W9-AHW-842

Dx/Rx:
Lymphoma

Daniel O. Persky, MD

Assistant Professor of Clinical Medicine
Arizona Cancer Center
Tuscon, AZ

Series Editor: Manish A. Shah, MD

Division of GI Oncology
Memorial Sloan-Kettering Cancer Center
New York, NY

JONES AND BARTLETT PUBLISHERS
Sudbury, Massachusetts
BOSTON   TORONTO   LONDON   SINGAPORE

World Headquarters
Jones and Bartlett Publishers
40 Tall Pine Drive
Sudbury, MA 01776
978-443-5000
info@jbpub.com
www.jbpub.com

Jones and Bartlett Publishers Canada
6339 Ormindale Way
Mississauga, Ontario L5V 1J2
Canada

Jones and Bartlett Publishers International
Barb House, Barb Mews
London W6 7PA
United Kingdom

Jones and Bartlett's books and products are available through most bookstores and online booksellers. To contact Jones and Bartlett Publishers directly, call 800-832-0034, fax 978-443-8000, or visit our website, www.jbpub.com.

Substantial discounts on bulk quantities of Jones and Bartlett's publications are available to corporations, professional associations, and other qualified organizations. For details and specific discount information, contact the special sales department at Jones and Bartlett via the above contact information or send an email to specialsales@jbpub.com.

The authors, editor, and publisher have made every effort to provide accurate information. However, they are not responsible for errors, omissions, or for any outcomes related to the use of the contents of this book and take no responsibility for the use of the products and procedures described. Treatments and side effects described in this book may not be applicable to all people; likewise, some people may require a dose or experience a side effect that is not described herein. Drugs and medical devices are discussed that may have limited availability controlled by the Food and Drug Administration (FDA) for use only in a research study or clinical trial. Research, clinical practice, and government regulations often change the accepted standard in this field. When consideration is being given to use of any drug in the clinical setting, the health care provider or reader is responsible for determining FDA status of the drug, reading the package insert, and reviewing prescribing information for the most up-to-date recommendations on dose, precautions, and contraindications, and determining the appropriate usage for the product. This is especially important in the case of drugs that are new or seldom used.

Library of Congress Cataloging-in-Publication Data
Persky, Daniel O.
    Dx/Rx. Lymphoma / Daniel O. Persky.
        p. ; cm. — (Jones and Bartlett publishers Dx/Rx oncology series)
    Includes bibliographical references and index.
    ISBN-13: 978-0-7637-5024-4
    ISBN-10: 0-7637-5024-7
    1. Lymphomas—Handbooks, manuals, etc. I. Title. II. Title: Lymphoma.
III. Series. [DNLM: I. Lymphoma—therapy—Handbooks. WH 39 P466d 2007]
    RC280.L9P47 2007
    616.99'446—dc22
    6048   200603644

Production Credits
Executive Publisher: Christopher Davis
Production Director: Amy Rose
Associate Editor: Kathy Richardson
Associate Production Editor: Amanda Clerkin
Marketing Manager: Katrina Gosek
Associate Marketing Manager:
    Rebecca Wasley
V.P. Manufacturing and Inventory
    Control: Therese Connell

Manufacturing and Inventory
    Control Supervisor: Amy Bacus
Composition: ATLIS Graphics
Cover Design: Anne Spencer
Cover Image: © Sebastian Kaulitzki/
    ShutterStock, Inc.
Printing and Binding: Courier Stoughton
Cover Printing: Courier Stoughton

Printed in the United States of America
11 10 09 08 07   10 9 8 7 6 5 4 3 2

Dedication

To my parents Raisa and Oskar Persky, and to my mentor
Craig H. Moskowitz, without whom this work would not be
possible.

Table of Contents

Editor's Preface

It is my pleasure to introduce the latest addition to the Dx/Rx Oncology Series—*Dx/Rx: Lymphoma*. This is an essential handbook for the practicing oncologist. The diagnosis and management of lymphoma is complicated by significant heterogeneity and complexity of the disease. This handbook does an excellent job of introducing the concept of clonal disorders of B and T cells, describes the variety of diseases that are encompassed within the realm of *lymphomas*, and goes into surprising, easy-to-read, detail about the diagnosis and treatment of the most common lymphoma sub-types, including *diffuse large B-cell lymphoma, follicular lymphoma, marginal zone* and *mantle cell lymphoma,* and of course *Hodgkin's lymphoma.* The book also has an incredibly informative and useful chapter summarizing the common chemotherapy regimens used for the management of lymphomas. This is a well written and easy-to-follow primer on the management of a complex and diverse group of diseases. I believe you will find this handbook, along with the others in the Dx/Rx Oncology series, invaluable!

Manish A. Shah, MD

CHAPTER 1

Overview

- Lymphomas are clonal disorders that arise from B or T cells, rarely NK cells.
- They are extremely heterogenous secondary to multiple histologic subtypes and variable clinical presentations.
- This heterogeneity has important prognostic implications and impacts on whether treatment is administered with curative intent.
- This will not be an exhaustive review of lymphomas. The focus of this chapter is twofold:
  - Understand the diagnosis, staging, and initial evaluation of a lymphoma patient
  - Know how to manage the most common lymphoid malignancies

■ Epidemiology

- Estimates by American Cancer Society for 2007:
  - Number of new cases:
    - Non-Hodgkin's lymphoma (NHL): 63,190
    - Hodgkin's lymphoma (HL): 8,190
  - Deaths: NHL 18,660; HL 1,070
  - Five percent of new cancer cases and 3% cancer deaths for 2007[1]
- Incidence has increased approximately twofold over the last 30 years. The cause is unclear, but the increase is most significant in elderly patients with aggressive lymphoma.
- Human immunodeficiency virus (HIV)-related lymphomas have begun to decline.
- Overall incidence increases with age; mean age at presentation is 65 years.
- Slight male predominance: 22.7 males and 15.9 females per 100,000 for 1996–2000 (for NHL)[2]

■ Geographical variability: More common in the United States and Europe than in Asia

■ Etiology and Risk Factors

■ Infections: HIV-1, Human T-lymphotropic virus type 1 (HTLV-1), Epstein-Barr virus (EBV), hepatitis C virus, Human herpesvirus 8 (HHV-8), *Helicobacter pylori, Borrelia burgdorferi* (*B. afzellii* species), *Campylobacter jejuni, Chlamydia psittaci*
■ Autoimmune diseases: Sjogren's syndrome, rheumatoid arthritis, systemic lupus erythematosus (SLE), polymyositis/dermatomyositis mixed cryoglobulinemia, celiac disease
■ Inflammatory: Crohn's disease
■ Immunodeficiency:
   • Acquired: HIV, medications for organ transplantation, and autoimmune disease treatment
   • Inherited: severe combined immunodeficiency, common variable immunodeficiency, Wiskott-Aldrich syndrome, ataxia-telangiectasia, hypogammaglobulinemia
■ Chemicals: herbicides (2,4-dichlorophenoxyacetic acid), organic solvents, possibly Agent Orange
■ Exposures: ultraviolet radiation

■ Presentation

■ Almost two-thirds of patients present with lymphadenopathy.
■ In aggressive and highly aggressive lymphomas, lymphadenopathy increases quickly; it waxes and wanes in indolent lymphomas.
■ "B" symptoms are present in up to 40%.
   • Defined as one of the following: fever greater than 38°C, drenching night sweats, or unexplained weight loss of greater than 10% of body weight over 6 months
   • Less common in indolent lymphomas
■ Up to one-third of patients may present with extranodal disease.
■ Infectious and inflammatory etiologies need to be ruled out:
   • Viral: EBV, cytomegalovirus (CMV), HIV
   • Bacterial: syphilis, tuberculosis, cat scratch disease
   • Parasitic: toxoplasmosis

* Inflammatory: sarcoidosis, SLE
* Medications: phenytoin, hydralazine, sulfa drugs
* Other cancers may also present with lymphadenopathy (see below).
  * Tender lymphadenopathy usually implies benign etiology.
* Generally, lymph nodes persistent for more than 2 weeks, greater than 1.5 cm in diameter, or smaller but growing in size will require an intervention.
  * If within 2 to 3 weeks there is no improvement, a biopsy should be considered.

■ Initial Evaluation

* Initial evaluation includes history, physical examination (including assessment of performance status according to ECOG/Zubrod scale[3] or Karnofsky[4] ranking [Tables 1-1 and 1-2]), complete blood count, electrolytes, liver function tests, lactate dehydrogenase (LDH), erythrocyte sedimentation rate if suspecting Hodgkin's lymphoma, calcium and uric acid if suspecting aggressive or highly aggressive lymphoma, of abdomen, pelvis and preferably chest, computerized tomography (CT) scanning with oral and intravenous contrast, and functional imaging (positron-emission tomography [PET]).

Table 1-1:   WHO/ECOG/Zubrod Performance Scale

0	Normal activity
1	Symptoms, but nearly fully ambulatory
2	Bedridden less than 50% of normal daytime
3	Bedridden more than 50% of normal daytime
4	Unable to get out of bed

Record what the patient is *capable* of.
Data from: Zubrod CG, Schneiderman M, Frei EI, Brindley C. Appraisal of methods for the study of chemotherapy of cancer in man: Comparative therapeutic trial of nitrogen mustard and triethylene thiophosphoramide. *J Chron Dis* 1960;11:7-33.

Table 1-2: Karnofsky Performance Status

Percent (%)	Criteria	Definition
100	No complaints, no evidence of disease	Able to carry on normal activity and to work. No special care is needed.
90	Normal activity; minor signs/symptoms of disease.	
80	Normal activity with effort; some signs or symptoms of disease.	
70	Cares for self. Unable to carry on normal activity or to do active work.	Unable to work. Able to live at home and care for most personal needs. A varying amount of assistance is needed.
60	Requires occasional assistance, but is able to care for most needs.	
50	Requires considerable assistance and frequent medical care.	
40	Disabled; requires special care and assistance.	Unable to care for self. Requires equivalent of institutional or hospital care. Disease may be progressing rapidly.
30	Severely disabled; hospitalization is indicated although death is not imminent.	
20	Very sick; hospitalization and active supportive treatment necessary.	
10	Moribund; fatal processes progressing rapidly.	
0	Dead	

Data from: Karnofsky DA, Ableman WH, Craver LF, Burchenal JH. The use of the nitrogen mustards in the palliative treatment of carcinoma. *Cancer* 1948;1:634-56.

- Subsequent workup should include Hepatitis B testing for B-cell lymphomas and functional imaging (PET scan) for some lymphoma types.
- HIV testing should be considered, particularly in Diffuse large B-cell lymphoma, Burkitt's lymphoma, and Hodgkin's lymphoma.
- Any organ-specific complaints must be evaluated for possible impairment by lymphoma, either by invasion or by mass effect.
- Bone marrow biopsy is done on nearly all patients. Cerebrospinal fluid (CSF) evaluation may be performed after the initial diagnosis, depending on the type and stage of lymphoma.

■ Making the Diagnosis

- After initial evaluation, proper histologic diagnosis and precise classification of the lymphoid neoplasm is the starting point for proper management.
- Adequate tissue volume is required.
  - Assessment of tissue architecture is critical. Replacement of normal architecture is seen in all lymphoid malignancies.
  - The lymph node has many compartments that are evaluated systematically.
  - A specific segment of the lymph node may be involved, as with marginal-zone lymphoma.
  - To allow for full assessment, an excisional biopsy is required to make the initial diagnosis of lymphoma. The specimen must be sent to the pathologist unfixed such that the proper tests can be run.
    - Cervical adenopathy may indicate metastatic head and neck cancer, particularly in patients with a smoking history.
      - An excisional biopsy in this setting could compromise a subsequent radical neck dissection; therefore, a fine-needle aspiration (FNA) biopsy is advantageous because it can exclude metastatic carcinoma.
      - Once a solid tumor is excluded, the node should be excised completely.

- If a patient has already been treated for a specific subtype of NHL and a relapse is suspected, then an FNA is acceptable to confirm recurrent disease.
- Mediastinal presentation in a patient younger than 40 years will most likely be Hodgkin's lymphoma or primary mediastinal large B cell lymphoma.
  - In this case, an open biopsy is not warranted and a mediastinoscopy or a Chamberlain procedure (anterior mediastinoscopy) is the procedure of choice.
- Patients who present with an abdominal mass will more likely have a solid tumor.
  - In this case, most patients can be diagnosed with a CT-guided core-needle biopsy.
  - If lymphoma is diagnosed on the frozen section, then multiple core biopsies will usually suffice to make an accurate diagnosis of the lymphoma subtype.
- Morphologic interpretation of cytology or tissue specimens is important, but not nearly as much as in the past. There are numerous causes of a misdiagnosis in lymphoma subtype, and an accurate diagnosis requires more sophisticated tests.
- Applying the classification for lymphoma requires integrating morphology with immunophenotyping by flow cytometry (fresh cells in suspension) and immunohistochemistry (IHC) (fixed tissue).
  - Immunophenotyping analysis is performed using a combination of both techniques.
  - Flow cytometry allows a large number of cells to be analyzed rapidly and with advanced gating techniques using multiple antibodies.
    - It can help to identify a small population of lymphoma cells in a complex specimen.
    - If negative for lymphoma, flow cytometry is not as helpful, because the tissue that was used may not have contained malignant elements by chance.
  - IHC helps to define architecture and identifying minor populations in a sample.
    - This is most important in delineating the Reed-Sternberg cell in Hodgkin's lymphoma.

- Diagnostic immunophenotyping analysis uses a panel of monoclonal antibodies. The abbreviation CD (cluster of differentiation) refers to a group of antibodies that recognize the same epitopes on the cell surface.
- Core-flow cytometric panels for the investigation of surface antigen expression are available. These panels can be specific for B or T cell malignancies (Table 1-3).
- The demonstration of chromosomal abnormalities can be performed using routine cytogenetics, in situ hybridization techniques, interphase fluorescent in-situ hybridization (FISH), or polymerase chain reaction (PCR). Only a limited number of distinct abnormalities are relevant to clinical practice (Table 1-4).
- Most laboratories use interphase FISH or PCR to demonstrate chromosomal abnormalities or numerical changes.
  - Interphase FISH with multicolor probes usually makes a diagnosis, but PCR is required for sensitivity in detecting minimal residual disease.
  - Antibody-based methods can also be useful in detecting genetic abnormalities.
    - Examples are cyclin D1 for mantle cell lymphoma and ALK-1 in anaplastic large cell lymphoma. Both of these lymphomas have a specific cytogenetic abnormality—t(11;14) and t(2;5), respectively.
- *The demonstration of monoclonality is diagnostic for lymphoma.*
- In most B cell lymphomas, monoclonality can be demonstrated using light chain restriction and flow cytometry.
- Flow cytometry for T cell lymphomas is difficult. PCR for T-cell receptor rearrangements is the technique of choice.

Table 1-3:   Determining Cell of Origin

Origin	Surface markers
B cell	CD 19, 20, 21, 22, 79a
T cell	CD 2, 3, 4, 7, 8
NK cell	CD 16, 56, 57

Table 1-4: Distinguishing Features of Lymphoma Subtypes

Lymphoma	Immunohistochemistry	Cytogenetics	Molecular
Follicular lymphoma	CD$_5$−, **CD$_{10}$+**, CD$_{20}$+, CD$_{23}$−, sIg+	t(14;18)	IgH/**bcl-2**
Marginal zone lymphoma	CD$_5$−, CD$_{10}$−, CD$_{20}$+, CD$_{23}$−, sIg+	Trisomy 3, t(11;18), t(14;18)	*API2/MALT1*, *IgH/MALT1*
Small lymphocytic lymphoma	CD$_5$+, CD$_{10}$−, CD$_{20}$dim+, CD$_{23}$+, FMC7−, **sIgdim+**	del 13q, del 11q, trisomy 12, del 17p	N/A
Mantle cell lymphoma	CD$_5$+, CD$_{10}$−, CD$_{20}$+, CD$_{23}$−, FMC7+, sIg+	t(11;14)	**cyclin D1**/IgH
Diffuse large B-cell lymphoma	CD$_5$−/+, CD$_{10}$−/+, CD$_{20}$+, sIg+	3q27 translocations (30%), t(14;18)(20%)	bcl-6, IgH/bcl-2
Burkitt's lymphoma	CD$_5$−, CD$_{10}$+, CD$_{20}$+, CD$_{23}$−, sIg+	t(8;14)	**c-myc**/IgH (**bcl-2−**)
Anaplastic large cell lymphoma (primary systemic)	CD$_{4}$+/−, CD$_{25}$+, **CD$_{30}$+**, EMA+/−, ALK+/−	t(2;5) (50%)	*NPM/ALK*
Hodgkin's lymphoma	CD$_{15}$+, CD$_{20}$−/+, **CD$_{30}$+**	N/A	N/A

Notes: Distinguishing characteristics are in **bold**, fusion genes are in *italics*, most common abnormalities are listed first. Morphologic appearance should be assessed first. Abbreviations: sIg = surface immunoglobulin; EMA = epithelial membrane antigen; ALK = anaplastic lymphoma kinase; N/A = not applicable. Chromosomal locations of genes: IgH−14, Igκ, Igλ, cyclin D1−11, bcl-2−18, bcl-6−3, c-myc−8.

* The absence of monoclonality should make the underlying diagnosis questionable, and a repeat biopsy will likely be necessary.

■ Classification

* Several classifications exist that were developed sequentially: Rappaport (1966),[5] Kiel (1974),[6] Lukes and Collins (1974),[7] Working Formulation (1982),[8] Revised European-American Classification (1994),[9] and the World Health Organization Classification (WHO) (1999).[10]
* Primary cutaneous lymphomas (ie, lymphomas confined to the skin) are now incorporated into the combined WHO/European Organization for Research and Treatment of Cancer classification.[11]
* The latest, most comprehensive classification is the WHO classification, developed by the International Lymphoma Study Group, initially formed in 1991 (Table 1-5).[10]
* The WHO classification is broken down by cell origin (B, T, or NK) and by cell maturity (precursor or mature).

Table 1-5: WHO Classification of Lymphoid Neoplasms

B-cell neoplasms
   Precursor B-cell neoplasm
      Precursor B-lymphoblastic leukemia/lymphoma (precursor B-cell acute lymphoblastic leukemia)
   Mature (peripheral) B-cell neoplasms*
      B-cell chronic lymphocytic leukemia/small lymphocytic lymphoma
      B-cell prolymphocytic leukemia
      Lymphoplasmacytic lymphoma
      Splenic marginal zone B-cell lymphoma (+/− villous lymphocytes)
      Hairy cell leukemia
      Plasma cell myeloma/plasmacytoma
      Extranodal marginal zone B-cell lymphoma of MALT type
      Nodal marginal zone B-cell lymphoma (+/- monocytoid B cells)
      Follicular lymphoma
      Mantle-cell lymphoma
      Diffuse large B-cell lymphoma
         Mediastinal large B-cell lymphoma
         Primary effusion lymphoma
      Burkitt's lymphoma/Burkitt cell leukemia

Table 1-5:   continued

T-cell and NK-cell neoplasms
  Precursor T-cell neoplasm
    Precursor T-lymphoblastic lymphoma/leukemia (precursor T-cell acute lymphoblastic leukemia)
  Mature (peripheral) T-cell neoplasms*
    T-cell prolymphocytic leukemia
    T-cell granular lymphocytic leukemia
    Aggressive NK-cell leukemia
    Adult T-cell lymphoma/leukemia (HTLV-1)
    Extranodal NK/T-cell lymphoma, nasal type
    Enteropathy-type T-cell lymphoma
    Hepatosplenic gamma-delta T-cell lymphoma
    Subcutaneous panniculitis-like T-cell lymphoma
    Mycosis fungoides/Sezary syndrome
    Anaplastic large-cell lymphoma, T/null cell, primary cutaneous type
    Peripheral T-cell lymphoma, not otherwise characterized
    Angioimmunoblastic T-cell lymphoma
    Anaplastic large-cell lymphoma, T/null cell, primary systemic type
Hodgkin's lymphoma (Hodgkin's disease)
  Nodular lymphocyte-predominant Hodgkin's lymphoma
  Classical Hodgkin's lymphoma
    Nodular sclerosis Hodgkin's lymphoma (grades 1 and 2)
    Lymphocyte-rich classical Hodgkin's lymphoma
    Mixed cellularity Hodgkin's lymphoma
    Lymphocyte depletion Hodgkin's lymphoma

Note: Only major categories are included. Common entities are shown in **bold.** *B- and T-/NK-cell neoplasms are grouped according to major clinical presentations (predominantly disseminated/leukemic, primary extranodal, predominantly nodal).
Abbreviations: HTLV1 +, human T-cell lymphotropic virus; MALT, mucosa-associated lymphoid tissue; NK, natural killer.
Data from: Harris NL, Jaffe ES, Diebold J, et al. World Health Organization classification of neoplastic diseases of the hematopoietic and lymphoid tissues: report of the Clinical Advisory Committee meeting-Airlie House, Virginia, November 1997. *J Clin Oncol* 1999;17(12):3835-49.

- The relative importance of clinical features, morphology, immunophenotype, and genetics differs according to lymphoma subtype and is difficult to remember (Table 1-6).[12]
- Lymphomas can be separated by clinical behavior (Table 1-7).[13]

Table 1-6: Presenting Features of Common B- and T-cell non-Hodgkin's Lymphomas

Lymphoma subtype	Frequency*	Age	Male	Stage I	II	III	IV	B	↑LDH	KPS <80	X	>1 EN	BM	IPI 0/1	2/3	4/5
Diffuse large B-cell	31	64	55	25	29	13	33	33	53	24	30	29	16	35	46	19
Follicular	22	59	42	18	15	16	51	28	30	9	28	23	42	45	48	7
Small lymphocytic lymphoma/chronic lymphocytic leukemia	6	65	53	4	5	8	83	33	41	11	13	29	72	23	64	13
Mantle cell	6	63	74	13	7	9	71	28	40	21	25	51	64	23	54	23
Peripheral T-cell	6	61	55	8	12	15	65	50	64	32	12	45	36	17	52	31
Mucosa-associated lymphoid tissue	5	60	48	39	28	2	31	19	27	15	8	31	14	44	48	8
Mediastinal large B-cell	2	37	34	10	56	3	31	38	81	22	52	19	3	52	37	11
Anaplastic large cell	2	34	69	19	32	10	39	53	45	26	17	28	13	61	18	21

* % of total cases. With the exception of median age at time of diagnosis, all numbers represent percent of patients with the listed feature

Abbreviations: B = B symptoms; >1 EN = more than one extranodal site involvement, including BM; BM = bone marrow involvement; GI = gastrointestinal tract involvement; IPI = international prognostic index; KPS <80 = Karnofsky performance scale less than 80%; ↑LDH = elevated lactate dehydrogenase; X = bulky disease over 10 cm in maximal diameter.

Modified with permission from Armitage JO, Weisenburger DD. New approach to classifying non-Hodgkin's lymphomas: clinical features of the major histologic subtypes. Non-Hodgkin's Lymphoma Classification Project. *J Clin Oncol* 1998;16(8):2780-95.

Table 1-7: **Classification of Most Common WHO Lymphoma Subtypes Based on Their Clinical Behavior**

Indolent:
    B-cell:
        Chronic lymphocytic leukemia/small lymphocytic lymphoma
        Follicular lymphoma (grades 1–3A)
        Hairy cell leukemia
        Marginal zone lymphoma
        Plasma cell myeloma
    T cell/NK cell:
        Mycosis fungoides
Aggressive:
    B cell:
        Follicular lymphoma grade 3B
        Mantle cell lymphoma
        Diffuse large B-cell lymphoma
    T cell/NK cell:
        Peripheral T-cell lymphoma, not otherwise specified
        Angioimmunoblastic T-cell lymphoma
        Anaplastic large-cell lymphoma
Highly aggressive:
    B-cell:
        Burkitt's lymphoma
        Precursor B-lymphoblastic lymphoma/leukemia
    T cell/NK cell:
        Precursor T-lymphoblastic lymphoma/leukemia

- Indolent: Grow over months; untreated patients live for years.
- Aggressive: grow over weeks; untreated patients live for months.
- Highly aggressive: grow over days; untreated patients live for weeks.

■ Staging

- Ann Arbor staging classification, modified at Cotswolds meeting in 1989 and initially used for Hodgkin's lymphoma, is also used for non-Hodgkin's lymphoma (Table 1-8).[14]
  - Note that patients with more than one extranodal contiguous extension site (E) should most properly be classified as stage IV, as opposed to stage IIEE, for example.

Table 1-8:   Ann Arbor Classification (modified at Cotswolds)

Stage	Presentation
I	Single lymph node region
II	Two or more lymph node regions on the same side of the diaphragm
III	Lymph node regions on both sides of the diaphragm
IV	Extralymphatic noncontiguous involvement

Suffixes:
B: "B" symptoms
A: Absence of "B" symptoms
E: Extralymphatic contiguous involvement (can be encompassed in the same radiation field)
X: Bulky (greater than 10 cm)
S: Splenic involvement

Modified with permission from Lister TA, Crowther D, Sutcliffe SB, et al. Report of a committee convened to discuss the evaluation and staging of patients with Hodgkin's disease: Cotswolds meeting. *J Clin Oncol* 1989;7(11):1630-6.

- The staging is not as important for indolent lymphomas, which usually present with advanced stage (III/IV) disease.
- To complete the staging:
  - Bone marrow biopsy
    - Involvement usually is focal.
    - Aspirate is less important, because it does not preserve the morphology and may miss lymphoma focus.
    - Bilateral biopsies increase the yield but change the stage in only a small number of patients.
    - Low yield in patients with limited stage (I/II) lymphoma.
  - CSF should be examined by lumbar tap in highly aggressive lymphomas (Burkitt and lymphoblastic) and in patients with aggressive lymphoma with an elevated LDH, advanced stage, and a poor performance status, in addition to patients with testicular and paranasal sinus involvement.

Table 1-9: IWC (Cheson) Response Criteria

Response category	Physical examination	Lymph nodes	Lymph node masses	Bone marrow
CR (complete response)	Normal	Normal	Normal	Normal
CRu (complete response, unconfirmed)	Normal	Normal	Normal	Indeterminate
	Normal	Normal	>75% decrease	Normal or indeterminate
PR (partial response)	Normal	Normal	Normal	Positive
	Normal	≥50% decrease	≥50% decrease	Irrelevant
	Decrease in liver/spleen	≥50% decrease	≥50% decrease	Irrelevant
POD (progression of disease)/ relapse	Enlarging liver/spleen, new sites	New or increased	New or increased	Reappearance

Data from: Cheson BD, Horning SJ, Coiffier B, et al. Report of an international workshop to standardize response criteria for non-Hodgkin's lymphomas. NCI Sponsored International Working Group. *J Clin Oncol* 1999; 17(4):1244.

■ Response Criteria

- International Working Group criteria, also known as Cheson criteria or IWC, are commonly used to evaluate response based on transverse diameter as well as on the sum of the products of the greatest diameters (Table 1-9).[15]
  - The criteria also define end points for clinical trials, such as progression-free survival and event-free survival (Table 1-10).

Table 1-10: Definitions of End Points for Clinical Trials (from Cheson)

End point	Response category	Definition	Point of measurement
Overall survival	All patients	Death from any cause	Trial entry
Event-free survival	All patients	Failure or death from any cause	Trial entry
Progression-free survival	All patients	Disease progression or death from any cause	Trial entry
Disease-free survival	CR, CRu	Time to relapse	First documentation of response
Response duration	CR, CRu, PR	Time to relapse or progression	First documentation of response
Time to progression	All patients	Time to progression or death related to lymphoma	Trial entry
Time to next treatment	All patients	Time when next treatment is needed	Trial entry
Lymphoma-specific survival	All patients	Death related to lymphoma	Death

Modified with permission from Cheson BD, Pfistner B, Juweid ME, et al. Revised response criteria for malignant lymphoma. *J Clin Oncol* 2007;25(5):579-86.

- The criteria are for NHL but commonly apply to HL as well.
- The criteria have recently been modified to incorporate PET scanning.
- Category of complete response (unconfirmed) [Cru] is eliminated.
- Category is stable disease (SD), where there is no response or progression, is introduced.
- Definition of other responses depends on whether the type of lymphoma is consistently PET-positive, or whether the PET scan was positive prior to therapy, versus variably PET-positive lymphoma, or negative PET scan prior to therapy.[14]

■ References

1. American Cancer Society. *Cancer Facts and Figures 2006.* Atlanta, GA: American Cancer Society.
2. Fisher RI, Mauch PM, Harris NL, Friedberg JW. Section 2: Non-Hodgkin's lymphomas. In: DeVita VT, Hellman S, Rosenberg SA, eds. *Cancer: Principles & Practice of Oncology.* 7th ed. Philadelphia, PA: Lippincott Williams & Wilkins; 2005:1957–1997.
3. ZuGrod CG, Schneiderman M, Frei EI, et al. Appraisal of methods for the study of chemotherapy of cancer in men: comparative therapeutic trial of nitrogen mustard and triethylene thiophosphoramide. *J Chron Dis.* 1960;11:7–33.
4. Karuofsky DA, Ableman WH, Crower LF, Burehenal JH. The use of the nitrogen mustards in the palliative treatment of carcinoma. *Cancer.* 1948;1:634–656.
5. Rappaport H. Tumors of the hematopoietic system. In: *Atlas of Tumor Pathology.* Washington, DC: US Armed Forces Institute of Pathology; 1966:sec 3, fasc 8.
6. Lennert K, Mohri M, Stein H, Kaiserling E. The histopathology of malignant lymphoma. *Br J Haematol.* 1975;31 (Suppl): 193–203.
7. Lukes RJ, Collins RD. Immunologic characterization of human malignant lymphomas. *Cancer.* 1974;34(4 Suppl): 1488–1503.
8. National Cancer Institute sponsored study of classifications of non-Hodgkin's lymphomas: summary and description of a working formulation for clinical usage. The Non-Hodgkin's

Lymphoma Pathologic Classification Project. *Cancer.* 1982;49(10):2112–2135.

9. Harris NL, Jaffe ES, Stein H, et al. A revised European-American classification of lymphoid neoplasms: a proposal from the International Lymphoma Study Group. *Blood.* 1994;84(5):1361–1392.

10. Harris NL, Jaffe ES, Diebold J, et al. World Health Organization classification of neoplastic diseases of the hematopoietic and lymphoid tissues: report of the Clinical Advisory Committee meeting–Airlie House, Virginia, November 1997. *J Clin Oncol.* 1999;17(12):3835–3849.

11. Willemze R, Jaffe ES, Burg G, et al. WHO-EORTC classification for cutaneous lymphomas. *Blood.* 2005;105(10): 3768–3785.

12. Armitage JO, Weisenburger DD. New approach to classifying non-Hodgkin's lymphomas: clinical features of the major histologic subtypes. Non-Hodgkin's Lymphoma Classification Project. *J Clin Oncol.* 1998;16(8):2780–2795.

13. Jaffe ES, Harris NL, Stein H, Vardiman JW. *World Health Organization Classification of Tumours: Pathology and Genetics of Tumours of Haematopoietic and Lymphoid Tissues.* Lyon: IARC Press; 2001.

14. Lister TA, Crowther D, Sutcliffe SB, et al. Report of a committee convened to discuss the evaluation and staging of patients with Hodgkin's disease: Cotswolds meeting. *J Clin Oncol.* 1989;7(11):1630–1636.

15. Cheson BD, Horning SJ, Coiffier B, et al. Report of an international workshop to standardize response criteria for non-Hodgkin's lymphomas. NCI Sponsored International Working Group. *J Clin Oncol.* 1999;17(4):1244–1253.

16. Cheson BD, Pfistner B, Juweid ME, et al. Revised response criteria for malignant lymphoma. *J Clin Oncol.* 2007;25(5): 579–586.

CHAPTER 2

Diffuse Large B-Cell Lymphoma

■ Epidemiology

■ Most common non-Hodgkin's lymphoma subtype (31%)[1]
■ A paradigm of aggressive lymphoma: grows quickly over a matter of weeks but is curable.
■ Other lymphoma subtypes most commonly transform to diffuse large B-cell lymphoma (DLBCL).

■ Presentation

■ Mean age of presentation is 64 years, slight male predominance (55%).
■ Lymph nodes grow over several weeks, often symptomatic.
■ One-third exhibit "B" symptoms at presentation.
■ One-third present with stage IV disease; only 20–25% present with stage I/IE disease.
■ Extranodal involvement is present in about 70%.
  ● Sites include gastrointestinal (GI) tract, breast, bone, nose and sinuses, parotids, salivary glands, and sanctuary sites (testis and central nervous system (CNS).
■ Small percentage has bone marrow involvement (16% in one large series).
■ Lactate dehydrogenase (LDH) is elevated in majority of patients.

■ Pathology

■ Morphology: large cells (nuclei twice the size of a small lymphocyte), prominent nucleoli, basophilic cytoplasm, diffuse growth pattern, proliferation fraction greater than 40% but less than 100%.
■ Morphologic variants:[2]

- Centroblastic: large noncleaved cells, oval to round vesicular nuclei, fine chromatin, two to four membrane-clinging nucleoli, little cytoplasm.
- Immunoblastic: more than 90% of the cells have prominent central nucleolus, abundant basophilic cytoplasm.
  - More common in immunosuppressed patients
- Anaplastic: cells look like those of anaplastic large cell lymphoma (which is of T or NK origin) and express CD30 like it does, but are derived from B cells.
  - Large blast-like cells, may have horseshoe-shaped or multiple nuclei, prominent nucleoli, abundant cytoplasm, or grow in a cohesive pattern
- T-cell/Histiocyte-rich large B-cell lymphoma: prominent background of T cells or histiocytes
  - Resemble Hodgkin's lymphoma (HL) but distinguished from it by more aggressive clinical course (disseminated disease, worse prognosis) and morphologically by dominance of cytotoxic (CD8 positive) T cells and histiocytes and absence of expanded meshworks of follicular dendritic cells
- Lymphomatoid granulomatosis: Epstein-Barr virus positive, with T-cell-rich background
  - Extensive necrosis, few atypical large B-cells, angiocentric or angioinvasive infiltrative pattern
  - Distinguished from nasal/angiocentric lymphoma by extranodal presentation involving lung, brain, or kidneys (as opposed to upper airways, skin, or GI tract)
- Immunophenotype
  - B-cell antigens (CD 19, 20, 22, 79a), CD45, monoclonal surface IgM
  - Usually CD5 negative; if positive, portends a worse prognosis
  - DLBCL is the first lymphoma to undergo gene expression profiling,[3] corroborated in a subsequent study by Rosenwald et al.[4] (Figure 2-1).
    - Two main phenotypes: germinal center origin and activated B-cell

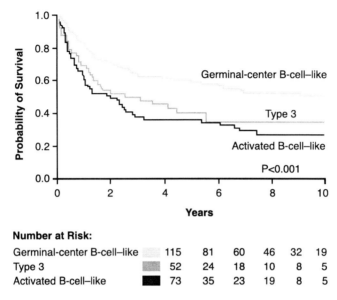

Figure 2-1: Kaplan–Meier estimates of overall survival of 240 previously untreated patients with diffuse large B-cell lymphoma according to the gene expression signature. Rosenwald et al. *NEJM.* 346(25):1937–1947, June 2002. Used with permission.

- Germinal center B-cell like (GCB): CD10 expression or bcl-6 expression with MUM1 negativity, better prognosis
- Activated B-cell like (ABC): bcl-2 and FLIP expression, worse prognosis
- "Type III": a third phenotype, poorly defined, worse prognosis
- Molecular classification was confirmed on immunohistochemistry,[5] based on CD10, bcl-6, and MUM1 antibody staining.
  - GCB: CD10 positive or CD10 negative/bcl-6 positive/MUM1 negative
  - ABC: CD10 negative/bcl-6 negative or CD10 negative/bcl-6 positive/MUM1 positive
- Cytogenetic and molecular changes:

- (14;18) translocations in 15–20% of the cases, versus 80–85% in follicular lymphoma
- Immunoglobulin variable regions rearranged
- Bcl-6 mutations or rearrangements

■ Prognosis

- International Prognostic Index (IPI) for aggressive NHL (Table 2-1)[6]; mnemonic *APLES*:
  - *A*ge older than 60 years
  - *P*erformance status (ECOG/Zubrod) greater than one
  - *L*DH greater than normal

Table 2-1: **International Prognostic Index (IPI) and Its Variations in Aggressive NHL**

Risk group	Number of risk factors	Percent patients in each group	5-year relapse-free survival (%)	5-year overall survival (%)*
International prognostic index				
Low	0–1	35	70	73
Low intermediate	2	27	50	51
High intermediate	3	22	49	43
High	4–5	16	40	26
Age-adjusted IPI, patients 60 years and younger*				
Low	0	22	86	83
Low intermediate	1	32	66	69
High intermediate	2	32	53	46
High	3	14	58	32

Table 2-1:   continued

Risk group	Number of risk factors	Percent patients in each group	5-year relapse-free survival (%)	5-year overall survival (%)*
Age-adjusted IPI, patients older than 60 years				
Low	0	18	46	56
Low intermediate	1	31	45	44
High intermediate	2	35	41	37
High	3	16	37	21
Second-line aaIPI			Four-year PFS (%)	Four-year OS (%)**
Low	0	13	70	74
Intermediate	1	27	39	49
High	2, 3	60	16	18
Stage-modified IPI			5-year PFS (%)	5-year OS (%)***
Low	0	24	94	97
Intermediate	1–2	66	79	77
High	3–4	10	60	58

*Data from: Anon. *NEJM* 1993.
**Data from: Hamlin et al, *Blood* 2003.
***Data from: Shenkier et al, *J Clin Oncol* 2002.

- Extranodal disease sites greater than one
- Stage (Ann Arbor/Cotswolds) III/IV
- IPI risk groups are based on the number of risk factors (above) present.
  - Zero or one, low risk; two, low-intermediate risk; three, high-intermediate risk; four or five, high risk
  - Overall survival (OS) for 5 years decreases from 71% to 51%, 43%, and to 26%, respectively.
  - IPI was developed before rituximab, but remains prognostic for rituximab-based therapy, although it's debatable if it still stratifies overall survival (OS) into four risk groups as well as before.[7]
- Age-adjusted IPI (aaIPI): IPI without age and extranodal sites (APLES without the vowels)
  - Patients older than 60 years have 5-year OS of 56% with low risk (zero factors), 44% with low-intermediate risk (one factor), 37% with high-intermediate risk (2 factors), 21% with high-risk (three factors) disease.
  - Patients 60 years or younger have 5-year OS of 83%, 69%, 46%, and 32%, respectively.
- At relapse prior to second-line treatment, age-adjusted IPI (sAAIPI) is prognostic.
  - sAAIPI stratified outcomes for second-line therapy with ICE (ifosfamide/carboplatin/etoposide) followed by high-dose therapy and autologous stem cell transplantation (HDT/ASCT) in a study of 150 patients.
    - Patients with zero risk factors had a 4-year OS of 74%; one risk factor, 49%; and two to three risk factors, 18%; 4-year progression-free survival (PFS) was 70%, 39%, and 16%, respectively.[8]
- Stage-adjusted IPI for limited stage (I/II) disease:
  - Age older than 60, LDH greater than normal, stage II, performance status greater than 1 (APLES without E, stage II instead of stage III/IV)
  - Ten-year OS was 90% (zero risk factors), 56% (one to two risk factors), and 48% (three to four risk factors) after three cycles of doxorubicin-based chemotherapy followed by involved field radiation therapy.[9]
- GCB patients had a 5-year OS of 76% as compared to 34% for non-GCB patients in the study by Hans et al.

that was mentioned earlier (5-year Event-Free Survival [EFS]: 63% vs. 36%).

■ It is unclear if GCB vs. non-GCB phenotype affects outcomes in patients undergoing ASCT or receiving rituximab: a study of relapsed/primary refractory patients from Memorial Sloan-Kettering suggested no effect of phenotype,[10] while a recent Dutch-Belgian study suggests that GCB phenotype had a superior outcome in poor-risk patients receiving ASCT as first-line therapy[11]; neither study incorporated rituximab.

   ● There is a suggestion that non-GCB phenotype benefits prefercutially from addition of rituximab to initial chemotherapy, but it is too early to tell whether rituximab should be withheld from anyone with DLBCL.

■ Gene expression profiles stratified outcomes based on 13 and 17 genes that did not overlap; a simplified model using six genes from both prior models remained predictive of outcome.

   ● BCL6, FN1, and LMO predicted better OS and BCL2; CCND2 and SCYA3 predicted worse OS.[12]

■ Individual studies identified expression of anti-apoptotic bcl-2 (particularly in non-GCB phenotype) and surviving; cell-cycle dysregulation-related changes such as mutated TP53 and expression of cyclin D2 and Skp2; expression of CD5; of transcription factors MUM1 and FOXP1; of angiogenesis markers sVEGF and endostatin; of pro-metastatic MMP9; high proliferative index (Ki67); decreased HLA class II molecule expression; and inability to handle oxidative stress as prognostically unfavorable. Expression of germinal center-related bcl-6, CD10, and HGAL; of CD21; and presence of tumor-infiltrating lymphocytes were prognostically favorable.

■ Negative positron-emission tomography (PET) scan at completion of therapy and in small studies as early as after first cycle of therapy predicts longer disease-free interval; incorporation of PET scanning in treatment stratification is being actively investigated.

   ● In a prospective trial of 90 patients, patients with a negative PET after 2 cycles of anthracycline-containing therapy achieved a higher complete remission (CR) rate, 2-year event-free survival (EFS), and 2-year OS.[13]

- Moskowitz and colleagues reported a phase II trial of 4 cycles of dose dense rituximab plus cyclophosha- mide, doxorubicin, and prednisone (R-CHOP) after which patients were restaged with a PET scan; those with uptake on PET underwent a biopsy of the most PET-avid site. Patients with a negative biopsy after PET and those with a negative PET proceeded to re- ceive 3 cycles of ICE, while those with a positive biopsy received 2 cycles of ICE, 1 of R-ICE, and then ASCT.
  - Only 13% of patients having a positive PET had a positive biopsy, obviating a need for upfront ASCT in most patients.
  - Patients with negative PET had a similar EFS to those with positive PET. [14]
- At this point PET scanning has a role in staging at di- agnosis and after completion of treatment (at least 3 weeks after completion of chemotherapy and 8–12 weeks after completion of radiotherapy), but its use for restaging during therapy remains investigational.

■ Treatment

Treatment of Early Stage (I/Nonbulky II) Disease

- The standard treatment is chemotherapy with CHOP- like regimen. It can be shortened from six to eight cycles to three cycles if followed by involved field radiation ther- apy (IFRT), particularly for patients with low-risk stage- adjusted IPI.
- In the past, nonbulky early stage disease was treated with radiation therapy alone. It had high relapse rate, mostly beyond the radiation field, and the treatment was largely abandoned.
- Subsequent early studies in the 1980s showed survival advantage of a combination of chemotherapy and radia- tion therapy.
- The landmark study by Miller et al.[15] randomized 200 patients to three cycles of CHOP every 3 weeks (CHOP- 21) followed by IFRT and 201 patients to eight cycles of CHOP (Figure 2-2).

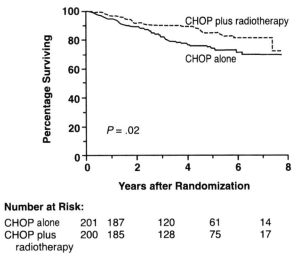

Figure 2-2: Overall survival of 201 patients receiving eight cycles of CHOP and 200 patients receiving three cycles of CHOP plus radiotherapy. There were 51 deaths in the CHOP-alone group, and 32 in the CHOP-plus-radiotherapy group. The estimated rates of survival at 5 years were 72% and 82% respectively. Miller et al., *NEJM*. 339(1):21–26, Figure 2, July 1998. Used with permission.

- Three cycles of CHOP plus IFRT were associated with better 5-year OS and PFS, largely benefitting patients older than 60 years.
- Ten-year follow-up showed that at 8 years the differences in OS and PFS between the two groups became statistically indistinguishable.
- Rituximab, chimeric (mouse humanized) anti-CD20 monoclonal IgG antibody is usually administered together with CHOP, mostly based on extrapolation of findings by Coiffier et al. for patients older than 60 years with advanced stage disease.
  - Miller et al added 4 infusions of rituximab to 3 cycles of CHOP followed by IFRT and compared it to historic cohort from the landmark study without rituximab.
    - 2-year OS was comparable: 95% with rituximab-containing therapy versus 93% without rituximab.

- 2-year PFS appeared better with rituximab: 94% vs. 85% without rituximab. [16]
- MInT trial, discussed below with advanced disease trials, enrolled patients younger than 60, with 73% of patients having stage I/II disease. It showed improvement in outcomes with addition of rituximab to 6 cycles of CHOP-like chemotherapy.

- The question of whether radiation therapy is truly necessary remains unresolved.
  - Eastern Cooperative Oncology Group 1,484 randomized 172 patients who obtained CR after eight cycles of CHOP to 30 cGy IFRT or observation, with the IFRT arm attaining 6-year disease-free survival of 73%, as opposed to 56% in observation arm ($P = .05$).[17]
    - No benefit for Failure-free survival (FFS) ($P = .06$ for the trend), time to progression, or OS was seen.
  - In a French study, LNH93-4, 576 patients older than 60 years were randomized to either four cycles of CHOP followed by 40 cGy IFRT or by observation.
    - No differences in outcome with a median follow-up of 6.8 years: 5-year EFS was 68% vs. 66%, and OS was 72% vs. 68% in CHOP and CHOP-IFRT arms, respectively.[18]
  - Another French study by Groupe d'Etude des Lymphomes de l'Adulte randomized 657 patients 60 years old and younger with aaIPI of 0 to three cycles of CHOP plus IFRT or to intensive chemotherapy with doxorubicin, cyclophosphamide, vindesine, bleomycin, and prednisone (ACVBP) followed sequentially by methotrexate, etoposide and ifosfamide, and cytarabine.
    - Patients in chemotherapy-only arm had better 5-year EFS (82% vs. 74%) and OS (90% vs. 81%) with median follow-up of 7.7 years.[19]
  - None of the above studies included rituximab.

Treatment of Advanced Stage (Bulky II/III/IV) Disease

- Chemotherapy with six to eight cycles of CHOP-like chemotherapy is the standard of care, with intrathecal methotrexate CNS prophylaxis for high-risk disease.

- CHOP and cyclophosphamide, vincristine, procarbazine, and prednisone (C-MOPP) were developed in the 1970s.
- Second- and third-generation regimens were developed in the late 1970s and 1980s by adding new agents and dose-intensification to improve CR and OS.
- Landmark study by Fisher et al.[20] randomized 897 patients to CHOP or one of three third-generation regimens: m-BACOD, ProMACE-CytaBOM, or MACOP-B. There was no significant difference in OS (45–46% at 5 years) and an increase in toxic deaths in third-generation regimens.
- Rituximab improved OS (70 vs. 57% at two years) and CR (76 vs. 63%) when added to eight cycles of CHOP in a French GELA study of 399 patients by Coiffier et al.[21] for patients older than 60 years with stage II–IV disease. The difference persisted in a recent 5-year update (Figure 2-3).
  - A similar U.S. Intergroup trial did not show a difference in OS due to interaction with rituximab maintenance randomization; in weighted analysis, addition of rituximab at any point improved OS.[22]
    - Intriguingly, bcl-6 negative patients accounted for most of the improvement in OS from R-CHOP in the Intergroup trial.[23]
  - Improvement was also seen in low-risk patients younger than 60 in MabThera International Trial (MInT), which actually had 73% of 823 patients with stage I/II disease.
    - With addition of rituximab to six cycles of a CHOP-like regimen, CR improved from 67% to 81%, 2-year time to treatment failure from 60% to 76%, and OS from 87% to 94%.[24]
- Radiation therapy: 30–40 Gy IFRT to bulky and extra-nodal sites is included in most of German studies, but generally not in U.S. or French studies.
- CHOP modifications:
  - CHOP can be administered with rituximab as above, it can be accelerated to every 2 weeks (CHOP-14) with growth factor support (G-CSF or GM-CSF), or it can include etoposide (CHOEP).
  - Pfreundschuh et al.[25,26] suggested that CHOP-14 resulted in better OS for patients older than 60, whereas CHOEP-14 or -21 benefited the younger group. Rituximab was not incorporated.

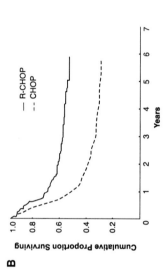

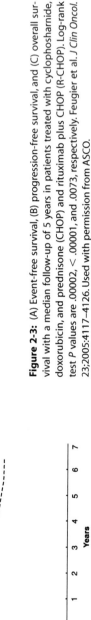

Figure 2-3: (A) Event-free survival, (B) progression-free survival, and (C) overall survival with a median follow-up of 5 years in patients treated with cyclophosphamide, doxorubicin, and prednisone (CHOP) and rituximab plus CHOP (R-CHOP). Log-rank test *P* values are .00002, < .00001, and .0073, respectively. Feugier et al. *J Clin Oncol.* 23;2005:4117–4126. Used with permission from ASCO.

- In a new study by Pfreundschuh and colleagues,[27] 828 elderly patients at all disease stages were randomized to six or eight cycles of CHOP with or without eight doses of rituximab.
  - Both rituximab arms had significantly improved EFS.
  - With median follow-up of 34.5 months, R-CHOP-14 for 6 cycles resulted in best 3 year OS of 78%, as compared to 68% in CHOP-14 for 6 cycles, 66% in CHOP-21 for 8 cycles, and 72% in R-CHOP-21 for 8 cycles; the difference in OS between CHOP-14 and R-CHOP-14 for 6 cycles was statistically significant (RR 0.63, p=0.003).
- HDT/ASCT in first CR has not been shown to improve survival and remains experimental.
  - A recent meta-analysis of 11 such trials confirmed lack of survival benefit and noted significant trial heterogeneity.[28]
- Prophylaxis of recurrence in CNS:
  - Intrathecal methotrexate, or less commonly cytarabine or high-dose systemic methotrexate
  - Prophylactic treatment is given if DLBCL involves a site with known propensity to relapse in CNS.
    - This is well established in cases of testicular and nasal sinus involvement; less so in cases of breast, ovarian, bone marrow, and extradural involvement.

Site-Specific Differences
- Testicular DLBCL:
  - One to 2% of all NHL
  - Lymphoma is the most common cancer to present with testicular mass in men older then 50 years; 80–90% of these lymphomas are DLBCL.
  - Presents usually with early-stage (IE/IIE) disease, median age 66.
  - High rate of extranodal relapse (including contralateral testis), over a third of those in CNS up to 10 years after presentation.[29]
  - The cells may have more plasmacytoid differentiation.
  - Higher frequency of chromosome 6q deletion.

- Prognosis may be worse stage for stage than for general DLBCL.
- Treated with unilateral orchiectomy of involved testis, anthracycline-containing chemotherapy such as CHOP, CNS prophylaxis, and low-dose radiation to contralateral testis to reduce the rate of relapse.

Treatment of Relapsed Disease

- Most relapses occur within first 2 to 3 years; rarely after 5 years.
- Salvage chemotherapy should be administered with the intent to proceed to high-dose chemoradiotherapy with autologous stem cell transplantation (HDT/ASCT), physiologic age permitting.
  - Regimens include ICE, DHAP, ESHAP, and mini-BEAM, now frequently combined with rituximab.
  - Infusional chemotherapy such as EPOCH or CDE may also be considered.
  - Addition of rituximab to ICE improved CR from 27% to 53% in 36 patients with relapsed/primary refractory disease.
    - Two-year PFS improved from 54% as compared to 43% in 147 historic controls, which was not statistically significant.[30]
- PARMA trial established the benefit of HDT/ASCT compared to conventional salvage chemotherapy (Figure 2-4).
  - Of 215 patients, 109 that responded to two cycles of DHAP were randomized to receive four more cycles or to undergo HDT/ASCT.
  - Five-year OS was 32% in conventional group and 53% in HDT/ASCT group.
  - Patients with IPI of 0 had similar OS with either treatment.
  - Treatment with HDT/ASCT abolished the prognostic importance of IPI.[31]
- Chemosensitivity is crucial in proceeding to HDT/ASCT and overcomes the adverse significance of primary refractory (as opposed to relapsed) disease.[32]
- Reduction of minimal residual disease may be advantageous.

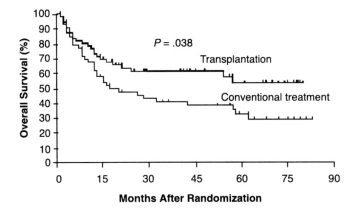

Figure 2-4: Kaplan–Meier curves for overall survival of patients in the transplantation and conventional-treatment groups. The data are based on an intention-to-treat analysis. Tick marks represent censored data. Philip et al., *NEJM*. 333(23):1540, Figure 2, 1995. Used with permission.

- A pilot study of four doses of rituximab at 6 weeks and 6 months after HDT/ASCT, with 25 of 35 patients with aggressive NHL having DLBCL showed 85% 2-year OS.[33]
- Tumor cells in the stem cell collection could contribute to relapse after HDT/ASCT.
- Allogeneic transplantation did not lead to improvement in OS compared to autologous transplantation, with significant treatment-related mortality that outweighed a lower relapse rate.[34]
  - Allo-transplant is often considered after relapse from auto-transplant but remains experimental in such settings.
    - A registry review of 114 such patients, including 44 with aggressive NHL, showed 1-year treatment-related mortality (TRM) of 22%, and 5-year OS and PFS of 24% and 5%, respectively, with greater benefit in patients in remission with good performance status and human leukocyte antigen-matched sibling donor.[35]

- Non-myeloablative ("mini-allo") transplantation may reduce TRM, but one of the largest studies by Morris et al. including 22 patients with DLBCL still showed 3-year TRM of 38%, with 3-year PFS and OS of 34%.[36]

■ DLBCL Variants

Primary Mediastinal Large B-cell Lymphoma (PMLBCL)

- One to 2% of NHL; 7% of DLBCL
- Patients are usually in their early 30s, slight female predominance.
- Often presents with superior vena cava syndrome and airway compromise
- Thought to originate from a thymic B-cell population
- Morphology shows large cells with clear cytoplasm and stromal sclerosis separating cells into nests.
- Unlike in regular DLBCL, bcl-6 and bcl-2 usually are not rearranged.
- Recent gene expression profiling study showed that PMLBCL shares features with classical HL, such as up-regulation of NFκB pathway genes.[37]
- Prognostic significance of germinal center phenotype probably cannot be applied to PMLBCL due to different cell origin and molecular profile.
- Lower expression of MHC class II genes remains an adverse prognostic factor.
- Treatment is with CHOP-like regimen combined with rituximab, followed by involved field radiation therapy to mediastinum for bulky disease.
  - More dose-dense/intense regimens may be helpful, such as CHOP-14 or doxorubicin/vincristine/cyclophosphamide (NHL-15), with an attempt to avoid mediastinal radiation.
- Survival is as good or better than for regular DLBCL (about 64–80% vs. 45–50% at 5 years)

Intravascular DLBCL

- Extremely rare: lymphoma cells in the lumina of small blood vessels

- The cells are large, with scant cytoplasm, large vesicular nuclei, and one or more nucleoli.
- May involve any organ, most commonly CNS and skin; lymphadenopathy uncommon
- Symptoms are due to organ disfunction and are nonspecific, so the diagnosis is often made late—up to half the cases are diagnosed at autopsy.
- In the largest series of 96 patients, median age was 67, diagnosis was established post-mortem in 16%, 91% had stage III or IV disease, 76% had "B" symptoms, 93% had elevated LDH, 82% had WHO performance status above 1, and 75% had high-risk IPI. Estimated 3-year OS was 27%.[38]
- The treatment is the same as in other DLBCL; there are not enough data to suggest otherwise.

General Treatment Approach
- Early stage DLBCL (I/nonbulky II):
  - Three cycles of R-CHOP-21 plus 30–40 Gy IFRT, or
  - Six to eight cycles of R-CHOP-21 (or R-CHOP-14 in patients older than 60 years)
- Advanced stage DLBCL (bulky II/III/IV):
  - Six to eight cycles of R-CHOP-21 (or R-CHOP-14 in patients older than 60 years)
  - Per most German protocols, 30–40 Gy IFRT to bulky sites may be considered.
- Relapsed DLBCL:
  - If good performance status, second-line regimen such as ICE, DHAP, ESHAP, or mini-BEAM, combined with rituximab
    - If sensitive to second-line regimen and transplant eligible, high-dose therapy and autologous stem cell transplantation (HDT/ASCT)
  - If poor KPS or refractory to second-line regimen, palliative chemotherapy (single-agent or combination)
  - CNS prophylaxis: at least four doses of intrathecal methotrexate for testicular and nasal sinus involvement; possibly also for breast, ovarian, bone marrow, and extradural involvement

■ References

1. Armitage JO, Weisenburger DD. New approach to classifying non-Hodgkin's lymphomas: clinical features of the major histologic subtypes. Non-Hodgkin's Lymphoma Classification Project. *J Clin Oncol.* 1998;16(8):2780–2795.

2. Harris NL, Jaffe ES, Diebold J, et al. World Health Organization classification of neoplastic diseases of the hematopoietic and lymphoid tissues: report of the Clinical Advisory Committee meeting—Airlie House, Virginia, November 1997. *J Clin Oncol.* 1999;17(12):3835–3849.

3. Alizadeh AA, Eisen MB, Davis RE, et al. Distinct types of diffuse large B-cell lymphoma identified by gene expression profiling. *Nature.* 2000;403(6769):503–511.

4. Rosenwald A, Wright G, Chan WC, et al. The use of molecular profiling to predict survival after chemotherapy for diffuse large-B-cell lymphoma. *N Engl J Med.* 2002;346(25): 1937–1947.

5. Hans CP, Weisenburger DD, Greiner TC, et al. Confirmation of the molecular classification of diffuse large B-cell lymphoma by immunohistochemistry using a tissue microarray. *Blood.* 2004;103(1):275–282.

6. A predictive model for aggressive non-Hodgkin's lymphoma. The International Non-Hodgkin's Lymphoma Prognostic Factors Project. *N Engl J Med.* 1993;329(14):987–994.

7. Sehn LH, Berry B, Chhanabhai M, et al. The revised International Prognostic Index (R-IPI) is a better predictor of outcome than the standard IPI for patients with DLBCL treated with R-CHOP. *Blood.* 2007; 109(5):1857–1961.

8. Hamlin PA, Zelenetz AD, Kewalramani T, et al. Age-adjusted International Prognostic Index predicts autologous stem cell transplantation outcome for patients with relapsed or primary refractory diffuse large B-cell lymphoma. *Blood.* 2003;102(6):1989–1996.

9. Shenkier TN, Voss N, Fairey R, et al. Brief chemotherapy and involved-region irradiation for limited-stage diffuse large-cell lymphoma: an 18-year experience from the British Columbia Cancer Agency. *J Clin Oncol.* 2002;20(1):197–204.

10. Moskowitz CH, Zelenetz AD, Kewalramani T, et al. Cell of origin, germinal center versus nongerminal center, determined by immunohistochemistry on tissue microarray, does not correlate with outcome in patients with relapsed and refractory DLBCL. *Blood.* 2005;106(10):3383–3385.

11. van Imhoff GW, Boerma EJ, van der Holt B, et al. Prognostic impact of germinal center-associated proteins and chromosomal breakpoints in poor-risk diffuse large B-cell lymphoma. *J Clin Oncol.* 2006;24(25):4135–4142.

12. Lossos IS, Czerwinski DK, Alizadeh AA, et al. Prediction of survival in diffuse large-B-cell lymphoma based on the expression of six genes. *N Engl J Med.* 2004;350(18):1828–1837.

13. Haioun C, Itti E, Rahmouni A, et al. [18F]fluoro-2-deoxy-D-glucose positron emission tomography (FDG-PET) in aggressive lymphoma: an early prognostic tool for predicting patient outcome. *Blood.* 2005;106(4):1376–1381.

14. Moskowitz CH, Hamlin PA, Horwitz SM, et al. Phase II Trial of Dose-Dense R-CHOP Followed by Risk-Adapted Consolidation with Either ICE or ICE and ASCT, Based upon the Results of Biopsy Confirmed Abnormal Interim Restaging PET Scan, Improves Outcome in Patients with Advanced Stage DLBCL. *Blood.* 2006; 108(11): 532a.

15. Miller TP, Dahlberg S, Cassady JR, et al. Chemotherapy alone compared with chemotherapy plus radiotherapy for localized intermediate- and high-grade non-Hodgkin's lymphoma. *N Engl J Med.* 1998;339(1):21–26.

16. Miller TP, Unger JM, Spier C, et al. Effect of Adding Rituximab to Three Cycles of CHOP Plus Involved-Field Radiotherapy for Limited-Stage Aggressive Diffuse B-Cell Lymphoma (SWOG-0014). *Blood.* 2004;104(11):158a.

17. Horning SJ, Weller E, Kim K, et al. Chemotherapy with or without radiotherapy in limited-stage diffuse aggressive non-Hodgkin's lymphoma: Eastern Cooperative Oncology Group study 1484. *J Clin Oncol.* 2004;22(15):3032–3038.

18. Bonnet C, Fillet G, Mounier N, et al. CHOP alone compared to CHOP plus radiotherapy for localized aggressive lymphoma in elderly patients: A study by the Groupe d'Etude des Lymphomes de l'Adulte. *J Clin Oncol.* 2007; 25(7):787–792.

19. Reyes F, Lepage E, Ganem G, et al. ACVBP versus CHOP plus radiotherapy for localized aggressive lymphoma. *N Engl J Med.* 2005;352(12):1197–1205.

20. Fisher RI, Gaynor ER, Dahlberg S, et al. Comparison of a standard regimen (CHOP) with three intensive chemotherapy regimens for advanced non-Hodgkin's lymphoma. *N Engl J Med.* 1993;328(14):1002–1006.

21. Coiffier B, Lepage E, Briere J, et al. CHOP chemotherapy plus rituximab compared with CHOP alone in elderly patients with diffuse large-B-cell lymphoma. *N Engl J Med.* 2002;346(4):235–242.

22. Habermann TM, Weller EA, Morrison VA, et al. Rituximab-CHOP versus CHOP alone or with maintenance rituximab in older patients with diffuse large B-cell lymphoma. *J Clin Oncol.* 2006;24(19):3121–3127.

23. Winter JN, Weller EA, Horning SJ, et al. Prognostic significance of Bcl-6 protein expression in DLBCL treated with CHOP or R-CHOP: a prospective correlative study. *Blood.* 2006;107(11):4207–4213.

24. Pfreundschuh M, Trumper L, Osterborg A, et al. CHOP-like chemotherapy plus rituximab versus CHOP-like chemotherapy alone in young patients with good-prognosis diffuse large-B-cell lymphoma: a randomised controlled trial by the MabThera International Trial (MInT) Group. *The Lancet Oncology.* 2006;7(5):379–391.

25. Pfreundschuh M, Trumper L, Kloess M, et al. Two-weekly or 3-weekly CHOP chemotherapy with or without etoposide for the treatment of elderly patients with aggressive lymphomas: results of the NHL-B2 trial of the DSHNHL. *Blood.* 2004;104(3):634–641.

26. Pfreundschuh M, Trumper L, Kloess M, et al. Two-weekly or 3-weekly CHOP chemotherapy with or without etoposide for the treatment of young patients with good-prognosis (normal LDH) aggressive lymphomas: results of the NHL-B1 trial of the DSHNHL. *Blood.* 2004;104(3):626–633.

27. Pfreundschuh M, Kloess M, Zeynalova S, et al. Six vs. Eight Cycles of Bi-Weekly CHOP-14 with or without Rituximab for Elderly Patients with Diffuse Large B-Cell Lymphoma (DLBCL): Results of the Completed RICOVER-60 Trial of the German High-Grade Non-Hodgkin Lymphoma Study Group (DSHNHL). *Blood.* 2006;108(11):205a.

28. Strehl J, Mey U, Glasmacher A, et al. High-dose chemotherapy followed by autologous stem cell transplantation as first-line therapy in aggressive non-Hodgkin's lymphoma: a meta-analysis. *Haematologica.* 2003;88(11):1304–1315.

29. Zucca E, Conconi A, Mughal TI, et al. Patterns of outcome and prognostic factors in primary large-cell lymphoma of the testis in a survey by the International Extranodal Lymphoma Study Group. *J Clin Oncol.* 2003;21(1):20–27.

30. Kewalramani T, Zelenetz AD, Nimer SD, et al. Rituximab and ICE as second-line therapy before autologous stem cell

transplantation for relapsed or primary refractory diffuse large B-cell lymphoma. *Blood.* 2004;103(10):3684–3688.

31. Philip T, Guglielmi C, Hagenbeek A, et al. Autologous bone marrow transplantation as compared with salvage chemotherapy in relapses of chemotherapy-sensitive non-Hodgkin's lymphoma. *N Engl J Med.* 1995;333(23): 1540–1545.

32. Kewalramani T, Zelenetz AD, Hedrick EE, et al. High-dose chemoradiotherapy and autologous stem cell transplantation for patients with primary refractory aggressive non-Hodgkin lymphoma: an intention-to-treat analysis. *Blood.* 2000;96(7): 2399–2404.

33. Horwitz SM, Negrin RS, Blume KG, et al. Rituximab as adjuvant to high-dose therapy and autologous hematopoietic cell transplantation for aggressive non-Hodgkin lymphoma. *Blood.* 2004;103(3):777–783.

34. Peniket AJ, Ruiz de Elvira MC, Taghipour G, et al. An EBMT registry matched study of allogeneic stem cell transplants for lymphoma: allogeneic transplantation is associated with a lower relapse rate but a higher procedure-related mortality rate than autologous transplantation. *Bone Marrow Transplantation.* 2003;31(8):667–678.

35. Freytes CO, Loberiza FR, Rizzo JD, et al. Myeloablative allogeneic hematopoietic stem cell transplantation in patients who experience relapse after autologous stem cell transplantation for lymphoma: a report of the International Bone Marrow Transplant Registry. *Blood.* 2004;104(12): 3797–3803.

36. Morris E, Thomson K, Craddock C, et al. Outcomes after alemtuzumab-containing reduced-intensity allogeneic transplantation regimen for relapsed and refractory non-Hodgkin lymphoma. *Blood* 2004;104(13):3865–3871.

37. Savage KJ, Monti S, Kutok JL, et al. The molecular signature of mediastinal large B-cell lymphoma differs from that of other diffuse large B-cell lymphomas and shares features with classical Hodgkin lymphoma. *Blood.* 2003;102(12): 3871–3879.

38. Murase T, Yamaguchi M, Suziki R, et al. Intravascular large B-cell lymphoma (IVLBCL); a clinicopathologic study of 96 patients with special references to the immunophemotypic heterogeneity of COS. *Blood.* 2007;109:478–485.

CHAPTER 3

Follicular Lymphoma

■ Epidemiology

- Most common indolent lymphoma (70%) and second most common non-Hodgkin's lymphoma (20%)
- A paradigm of indolent lymphoma: not curable, median survival 8-10 years, with suggestion of improving survival with rituximab-based treatment[1]
- Median age of onset about 60, slight female predominance, more common in the United States and Europe

■ Presentation

- Painless, diffuse, small lymphadenopathy
- Waxes and wanes over months to years; this varies widely from patient to patient.
- Spontaneous regressions occur, but usually are not durable.
- B symptoms only in about 20%
- Bone marrow involvement in 60–70%, usually paratrabecular
- Advanced stage (III/IV) at presentation in about 70%

■ Pathology

- Resemble normal germinal centers of secondary lymphoid follicles
- Differ from benign reactive follicular hyperplasia (RFH) in that the follicles in follicular lymphoma (FL) have higher density, lack internal polarity, and have monotonous appearance
- Interfollicular areas mostly contain tight meshworks of follicular dendritic cells and some T cells, but often have neoplastic cells as well.

- Mixture of centrocytes (small cleaved follicular-center cells) and centroblasts (large noncleaved follicular-center cells)
- The higher the proportion of centroblasts, the higher the grading and the aggressiveness of FL. The grading, by Mann and Berard,[2] is:
  - Grade 1: 0–5 centroblasts per high-power field
  - Grade 2: 6–15 centroblasts per high-power field
  - Grade 3: More than 15 centroblasts per high-power field
    - 3A: More than 15 centroblasts, but centrocytes still present
    - 3B: Centroblasts form solid sheets without residual centrocytes.
  - Grade 1 is the most common grade.
  - A diffuse large B-cell lymphoma (DLBCL) component can be associated with FL; percentage of diffuse component should be indicated.
  - The grading by Mann and Berard predicted FFS better than three other grading methods, but all four predicted overall survival (OS).[3]

Immunophenotype

- B-cell antigens (CD 19, 20, 22, 79a), monoclonal surface immunoglobulins (IgM 50–60%, 40% IgG, rare IgA)
- CD10 positive (60%), CD5 negative, CD43 negative, CD11c negative
- Strong cytoplasmic staining for bcl-2 distinguishes FL from RFH, which is bcl-2 negative.
- Interfollicular areas often stain for CD10 and nuclear bcl-6, unlike RFH.
- Lower MIB-1 (Ki-67) proliferation index than RFH or aggressive lymphomas

Cytogenetic and Molecular Changes

- Immunoglobulin genes rearranged, variable regions underwent somatic mutations
- t(14;18) (q32;q21) found in 80–85% of cases
  - The translocation juxtaposes Ig heavy-chain locus on chromosome 14 and bcl-2 locus on chromosome 18.

The IgH locus activates transcription of bcl-2, which blocks apoptosis.

▪ Additional cytogenetic abnormalities are almost always present at diagnosis, usually chromosomal additions or deletions, not translocations.

▪ Normal individuals also may have t(14;18); thus, the translocation can be used to confirm the diagnosis, but cannot be a sole basis for it.

▪ Several gene-expression-profiling studies have been performed:

 • One showed-regulation genes involved in cell cycle control, DNA synthesis, and increased metabolism.[4]

 • Another demonstrated significance of tumor infiltrating cells—the group with up-regulation of T-cell cell restricted genes ("immune response-1") had better survival than the group with up-regulation of genes expressed in monocytes and/or dendritic cells ("immune response-2").[5]

▪ Based on cytogenetic and molecular evidence, there seem to be at least two FL subgroups:

 • The larger subgroup progresses slowly, perhaps more due to impaired apoptosis than to actual growth; accumulates cytogenetic abnormalities; and transforms to DLBCL at a slow rate of 2–3% a year.

 • The other, smaller subgroup, more aligned with "immune response-2," grows more aggressively, is less responsive to chemotherapy, and transforms more rapidly.

Grade 3 FL

▪ It remains controversial:

 • whether grade 3 FL is clinically more similar to other FL or to DBLCL.

 • whether grade 3A is clinically different from grade 3B, with respect to the question above.

▪ Most studies show no difference in long-term OS curves between the three grades of FL, especially if low-stage patients, who have a better OS, are excluded. Considerable variation is caused by differences in pathologic subtyping, with older studies treating grade 3 as one entity.

- There is evidence of immunophenotypic, but not clinical, differences between grade 3A and 3B. In the study by Ott et al.:[6]
  - FL grade 3B was CD10 positive only 50% of the time, compared to 97–100% in grades 1–3A, and had plasmacytoid differentiation in 44%.
  - Grade 3B also had lower frequency of t(14;18) and higher frequency of chromosomal breaks at 3q27 involving BCL6 (possibly due to harboring a DLBCL component).
- Cases with greater than 50% of DLBCL component in the FL specimen have inferior survival; DLBCL component should be addressed separately from the FL grade.[7]
- Overall, grade 3B FL is treated like DLBCL with evidence of long-term remissions with anthracycline-based cyclophosphamide, doxorubicin, and prednisone (CHOP-like) therapy, whereas grade 3A may be treated similarly to grades 1–2 (if there is doubt, R-CHOP is acceptable in either case).

■ Variants

Cutaneous FL

- Rare, often involves the scalp
- Lower frequency of t(14;18) and bcl-2, but most express CD10 and bcl-6
- Tend to stay localized and can be treated with local therapy

Diffuse Follicle Center Lymphoma

- Mostly centrocytes in a completely diffuse pattern
- May maintain vaguely follicular appearance on close inspection
- Both centrocytes and centroblasts need to be of follicular center origin. Therefore, co-expression of CD10 and bcl-6 and evidence of t(14;18) are needed for diagnosis.
- Clinical outcomes are not well understood.

■ Prognosis

- Individual studies have shown that over-expression of anti-apoptotic bcl-2 and bcl-X_L, expression of MDM2 (signaling loss of p53 function), monocytoid B-cell differentiation, increased intrafollicular proliferative rate, increased diffuse areas, increased lymphoma-associated macrophage content, lower number of CD4 positive and of perifollicular FOXP3 cells are unfavorable.

- Expression of bcl-6 and CD10, consistent with germinal center phenotype, increased small vessel density, and high expression of cyclin B1, consistent with better response to CHOP, are favorable.
- Only 7% of FL patients have high-risk International Prognostic Index (IPI) of 4 or 5. This group has a median survival of 1 year.
- A Follicular Lymphoma International Prognostic Index (FLIPI) (Table 3-1) recently was proposed that stratifies patients more evenly than IPI (Figure 3-1).[8]
  - Five risk factors: (1) older than 60 years, (2) advanced stage (III/IV), (3) hemoglobin less than 12, (4) elevated LDH, and (5) more that four nodal sites of involvement–the memonic is NoLASH.
  - Nodal sites are cervical, axillary, mediastinal, mesenteric/celiac, para-aortic/iliac, inguinal (also epitrochlear and popliteal); bilateral involvement counts as two sites.
  - Zero or one risk factor (36% of the patients): 71% 10-year OS
  - Two risk factors (37% of the patients): 51% 10-year OS
  - Three to five risk factors (27% of the patients): 36% 10-year OS

Table 3-1: Follicular Lymphoma International Prognostic Index (FLIPI)

Risk group	Number of risk factors	Percent patients in each group	5-year OS (%)	10-year OS (%)
Low	0–1	36	91	71
Intermediate	2	37	78	51
High	3–5	27	52	36

Adapted with permission from Blood, Journal of the American Society of Hematology. Solal-Celigny, P., 2004, Vol. 104: 1258–1265

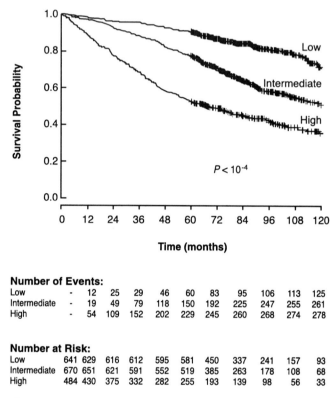

Number of Events:

Low	-	12	25	29	46	60	83	95	106	113	125
Intermediate	-	19	49	79	118	150	192	225	247	255	261
High	-	54	109	152	202	229	245	260	268	274	278

Number at Risk:

Low	641	629	616	612	595	581	450	337	241	157	93
Intermediate	670	651	621	591	552	519	385	263	178	108	68
High	484	430	375	332	282	255	193	139	98	56	33

Figure 3-1: Survival of the 1,795 patients according to risk group as defined by the Follicular Lymphoma International Prognostic Index. Used with permission from *Blood*, Journal of the American Society of Hematology. Solal-Celigny, P., 2004, Vol. 104: 1258–1265.

- FLIPI was defined in a pre-rituximab treatment cohort; the significance of FLIPI was recently confirmed in a group of 362 patients randomized to R-CHOP in a prospective trial, with significant difference in 2-year time to treatment failure (TTTF) between those with three to five risk factors (high risk) and those with less than three risk factors (low and intermediate risk).[9]
  - Stratification into three risk groups was seen if the groups were redefined as 1-2, 3, or 4-5 risk factors.

■ Transformation

* FL transforms to DLBCL at a rate of 2–10% a year independent of treatment strategy.
* Associated with p53 mutations, upregulated MYC expression, trisomy 7, 6q-, gain of 12q13–14, loss of p16
* Presents with rapidly growing lymphadenopathy and systemic symptoms
    * Splenic lesions in FL are suspicious for DLBCL transformation.
* Treatment is targeted at the most aggressive component, DLBCL.
* Even if DLBCL is cured, FL eventually relapses.
* Prognosis, as compared to de novo DLBCL, is controversial.
    * Earlier studies indicated widely disparate survival between 2.5 and 22 months, with most in 7–12 month range.
    * Recent review from St. Bart's hospital in London showed median survival of 1.2 years.[10]
    * As per the review above, 6/13 patients achieving complete remission after treatment of transformed disease attained survivals of more than 5 years.

■ Treatment

Treatment of Early Stage (I/II) Disease

* The only time FL is potentially curable (with radiation therapy [RT]), except for allogeneic transplantation.
* Radiation therapy (typically involved field radiation therapy [IFRT]) alone results in 40–45% freedom from treatment failure at 10 years in all published series, with median survival 12–15 years and 2% relapse after 15 years.
    * After RT, most patients relapse with limited disease, typically just outside the radiation field, and about 20% have long-term survival.
    * IFRT, 30-40 Gy, is the most commonly accepted treatment option for early stage FL.
* "Watch-and-wait" approach pioneered at Stanford showed that in a selected group of patients treatment

could be deferred until indications are met (see Groupe d'Etude des Lymphomes Folliculaires [GELF] criteria for treatment of advanced disease below).

- Ten-year OS was 85% in a retrospective series of 43 patients.
- At median follow-up of 86 months, 63% of the patients had not received treatment.[11]

■ Addition of chemotherapy:
- Addition of COP-Bleo or CHOP-Bleo (bleomycin) to IFRT by MD Anderson group[12] showed improved FFS but a 10-year OS of 82% comparable to historic control.
- Addition of chlorambucil to radiation did not affect FFS or OS.
- Randomized trial of IFRT vs. combined modality treatment is ongoing.

Treatment of Advanced Stage (Bulky II/III/IV) Disease

■ Disease usually relapses after first treatment, with each subsequent remission being shorter and each response rate decreasing.
- In 212 patients with FL (73% stages III/IV) treated with older regimens, median survival was 9 years, 4.5 years after relapse.
- Overall response rate decreased from 88% with first treatment to 48% with fourth treatment.
- Response duration decreased from a median of 31 months with first treatment to 13 months with second and third treatment, and 6 months with fourth treatment.[13]

■ Because therapy does not change OS, the key is deciding when to treat and to choose regimens with acceptable efficacy and toxicity.

■ Watch and wait—the safety of observation as initial approach was established at Stanford by Horning and Rosenberg.[14]
- Initial observation of 83 patients with low-grade NHL
- A 73% 10-year OS was seen, with median time to treatment of 3 years and spontaneous regression in 23%.

- No change in the risk or time to transformation was seen.
- Randomized trials confirmed that treating asymptomatic patients does not alter survival, although the trials used older regimens without rituximab.
  - A sample of 309 patients was randomized to observation vs. chlorambucil, with no difference in overall or disease-specific survival.[15]
    - Forty percent of patients older than 70 years did not require treatment at 10 years.
  - Eighty-nine patients were randomized to observation vs. intensive regimen with ProMACE-MOPP and 24 Gy TLI (total lymphoid irradiation).
    - Lower CR was seen in patients crossing over from observation to treatment arm (43% vs. 78%).
    - Improved 4-year DFS (51% vs. 12%), but no difference in 5-year OS of over 75%.[16]
  - One hundred ninety-three patients randomized to observation, prednimustine, or interferon alpha did not have a significant difference in OS (this study also established the GELF criteria mentioned below).
- Treatment criteria: best known are the GELF criteria,[17] which estimate disease burden:
  - Three or more lymph nodes sites greater than 3 cm in diameter
  - A single lymph node or extranodal site greater than 7 cm in diameter
  - Cytopenia: platelets less than $100,000/\mu L$ or absolute neutrophil count less than $1,000/\mu L$
  - Leukemic phase: circulating lymphoma cells greater than $5,000/\mu L$
  - Systemic symptoms
  - Marked splenomegaly, pleural effusion, ascites, or compressive symptoms (e.g., ureteral, spinal)
- There is a great variety of approaches with no standard of care.

- Most treatment options incorporate chemotherapy (with immunotherapy).
  - Other options include chemotherapy with radioimmunotherapy (RIT) or single-agent immunotherapy (rituximab).
  - Experimental approaches include vaccines and proteasome inhibitors (bortezomib).
- Radiation therapy alone:
  - Used in minimal stage III disease to prolong relapse-free survival in older studies
  - Could be used in locally advanced lesions for symptom control, if systemic disease does not require treatment
  - Not a good option for systemic treatment
- Combined modality therapy: adding radiation after chemotherapy
  - ProMACE-MOPP followed by TLI did not improve OS when compared to initial observation, as described above.
  - Although alkylators are known to cause MDS/AML (myelodysplastic syndrome or secondary acute myelogenous leukemia), when followed by low-dose total body irradiation (TBI) they resulted in 17% incidence of MDS/AML at 15 years in a cohort of 61 patients.[18]
  - Rarely used
- Chemotherapy approaches include:
  - Single agent vs. multiagent chemotherapy
  - Alkylator-based (CVP), anthracycline-based (CHOP), or purine analog-based (fludarabine) chemotherapy
  - Lower intensity (single-agent alkylator, CVP) vs. higher intensity (anthracycline-based, usually multiagent—CHOP, M-BACOD, ProMACE-MOPP) chemotherapy
- Single-agent alkylators: chlorambucil, cyclophosphamide
  - CR 30–66%, mean duration of response 2.5–4 years, slower achievement of CR than with multiagent therapy (12 vs. 5 months for CVP in an 1981 study), but no differences in outcomes
  - Trial with 228 patients randomized to receive oral cyclophosphamide vs. CHOP–Bleo showed no differ-

ence in CR (66% vs. 60%), TTTF (25% vs. 33% at 10 years), or OS (44% vs. 46% at 10 years).[19]

- Unplanned subgroup analysis showed better outcomes with CHOP-Bleo for follicular mixed lymphoma (roughly corresponding to current grade 2 FL); this contradicted the results of a prior randomized trial for this subgroup.

- Multiagent alkylator chemotherapy: CVP (cyclophosphamide, vincristine, prednisone)
  - One of most frequently used initial treatments for FL, studied for over 40 years
  - CR in the same 30–70% range, well tolerated
  - Note that modern studies quote much lower CR rates of 7–10%, possibly due to more stringent and standardized CR criteria and better imaging.
- Anthracyclines: doxorubicin, mitoxantrone—used in combinations, not as single agents
- Multiagent anthracycline chemotherapy: CHOP, Pro-MACE-MOPP
  - CR 35-70%; OS same as for cyclophosphamide and CVP
  - Generally preferred for FL grade 3
- Single-agent purine analogs: fludarabine, cladribine
  - Fludarabine: CR 37% in untreated, 18% relapsed FL
  - Significant hematotoxicity and infectious complications, with prolonged bone marrow suppression particularly prominent in older patients
  - Fludarabine vs. CVP:
    - In untreated FL, 5-year OS was similar (65% vs. 56% in the watch and wait cohort, 76% vs 62% in the immediate treatment cohort), with no significant difference in TTTF or time to progression.[20]
    - In relapsed FL, median OS was similar (57 vs. 44 months), but fludarabine treatment resulted in slightly improved progression-free survival (PFS) (11 vs. 9 months, $P=.03$).[21]
  - Cladribine (2-CdA): relapsed: CR 20%, response duration 5 months[22]
- Multiagent purine analog therapy: FC, FN, FND

- Fludarabine, cyclophosphamide: 60% CR in un-treated patients, small study[23]; was too toxic in a phase III study vs. CVP.
- Fludarabine, mitoxantrone: 44% CR, 88% 4-year OS in untreated patients[24]
- Fludarabine, mitoxantrone, dexamethasone: CR 47%, median failure-free survival 14 months in relapsed patients[25]
- Immunotherapy: interferon alpha (IFN)
    - Single-agent 17% CR, short duration
    - In combination with chemotherapy prolongs PFS but not OS
    - However, in the largest randomized trial of 571 patients (86% with FL, others with small lymphocytic lymphoma (SLL), IFN with six to eight cycles of anthracycline-based ProMACE-MOPP did not show significant differences in PFS (4.1 vs. 3.2 years) and OS (78% vs. 77% at 5 years).[26]
    - Meta-analysis of 10 phase III trials of 1,992 newly diagnosed patients showed a survival advantage to IFN of 6% at 10 years, which was more pronounced with higher IFN doses and intensive initial chemotherapy.[27]
        - The limitations are the heterogeneity of trials and lack of therapies incorporating rituximab (as well as of RIT and fludarabine).
    - Not often used in the United States because of toxicity and prolonged subcutaneous administration
- Immunotherapy: rituximab
    - Pivotal trial of 166 patients with indolent lymphoma treated with at least two prior regimens showed 48% response rate with median time to progression of 13 months and minimal side effects.[28]
    - Sixty-two untreated patients (71% stages III/IV) had 73% overall respose rate (ORR) and 37% CR at the 6-month reevaluation, with median PFS of 30 months.[29]
    - In a study of 58 patients, retreatment with rituximab showed ORR 40%, CR 11%, with median time to progression of 18 months.[30]

* Rituximab is now a frequently employed option in patients with lower tumor burden who still meet treatment criteria or/and with significant comorbidities precluding chemotherapy.
* Rituximab maintenance: new evidence of survival improvement
  * After completion of one treatment with four weekly doses, maintenance improved median event free survival from 12 to 23 months (P=.024) for all patients and from 19 to 36 months in patients with no prior chemotherapy (P=.009).[31]
    * The maintenance schedule was four cycles of one dose every 2 months.
  * In a phase II trial of maintenance vs. treatment at the time of progression, PFS was longer in the maintenance arm (31 vs. 7 months), but there was no difference in duration of efficacy of rituximab (31 vs. 27 months) or OS (72% vs. 68% at 3 years).[32]
    * The maintenance schedule was four weekly doses every 6 months for 2 years.
    * More patients in maintenance group were in CR.
  * Rituximab maintenance (four doses q6 months for 2 years) after CVP: in 237 newly diagnosed patients, 4.5-year PFS improved from 33% to 56% (P=NS) and 4.5-year OS from 72% to 88% (P=.03).[33]
    * Rituximab was not given with CVP, which would probably be done in practice now, limiting the applicability of this study.
  * Rituximab maintenance (1 dose q3 months for 2 years) after six cycles of R-CHOP-21 in first or second relapse: median PFS improved from 15 to 52 months, 3-year OS improved from 77% to 85% (P=.01) in a study of 465 rituximab-naïve patients.[34]
  * FL patients responding to rituximab had median rituximab concentration of 25μg/ml (as opposed to 6 μg/ml in nonresponders).[35] Subsequent pharmacokinetic studies indicated that such concentrations are achieved with a dose being given every 3 months (the study had 18/31 patients with FL).[36]

- ■ Therefore, it would seem most effective to use rituximab maintenance regimens where a dose is
given every 2–4 months, such as with Ghielmini's
or van Oers' schedules.
■ Chemoimmunotherapy: adding rituximab to chemotherapy prolongs TTTF, possibly increases OS.
  - ● CHOP vs. R-CHOP: in 428 untreated patients with
  subsequent randomization of IFN vs. autologous stem
  cell transplantation (ASCT), both TTTF and OS improved with median follow-up of 18 months. (2-year
  OS 90% vs. 95%).[37]
  - ● CVP vs. R-CVP: untreated patients received eight cycles, with significant improvement in CR from 10% to
  41%, median TTTF from 7 to 27 months, median time
  to progression from 15 to 32 months ($P<.0001$ for
  all), without significant OS change (Figure 3-2).[38]

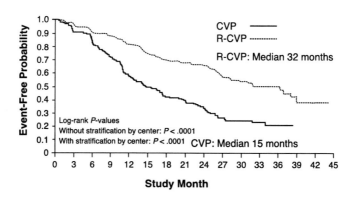

Study Month

Number at Risk:

CVP
159 140 129 109 87 75 64 58 46 28 21 12 5 0 0 0

R-CVP
162 156 144 140 131 119 111 106 95 68 50 32 20 10 2 0

Figure 3-2: Time to disease progression, relapse, or death after a median
follow-up of 30 months among 321 patients assigned to chemotherapy
with CVP or with R-CVP. Used with permission from *Blood,* Journal of the
American Society of Hematology. Marcus, R., 2005, Vol. 105: 1417–1423.

- If SD at cycle 4 was not considered failure, TTTF would be 15 months for CVP, comparable to other studies.
- Almost 50% of patients had poor-risk FLIPI .
- FCM vs. R-FCM: in relapsed patients after four cycles or therapy, CR improved from 23% to 40%, PFS from 21 months to not being reached at 3 years ($P=.0139$), 2-year OS from 70% to 90% ($P=.0943$).[39]
  - Of note, second randomization to rituximab maintenance (four weekly doses at 3 and 9 months) noted response prolongation (not reached vs. 26 months, $P=.035$).[40]
- Minimal residual disease:
  - Rituximab after CHOP improves the rate at which polymerase chain reaction (PCR) for t(14;18) becomes negative, which predicts for prolonged disease-free survival.
  - Patients responding to CHOP but still PCR positive received four weekly doses of rituximab.
  - Five-year freedom from relapse was 64% for PCR negative after CHOP with or without subsequent rituximab and 32% for PCR-positive patients (persistent or reverted to PCR positivity).[41]
- RIT
  - Radiation emitter conjugated to anti-CD20 antibody delivers targeted radiation with beneficial bystander killing while having limited tissue toxicity.
  - Two agents: Ibritumomab tiuxetan (Zevalin), a high-energy beta-emitter Yttrium-90 conjugated to the mouse "parent" antibody of rituximab, and Tositumomab/Iodine I_{131} Tositumomab (Bexxar), a lower energy beta and gamma emitter Iodine-131 conjugated to a mouse monoclonal IgG anti-CD20 antibody
  - Causes delayed myelosuppression at weeks 7–9
  - Not for patients with over 25% bone marrow involvement, because this causes unacceptable bone marrow suppression.
    - Zevalin: minimum 15% cellularity of the sample
    - Bexxar: 25% of intertrabecular space involvement, no cellularity requirement

- Zevalin: pivotal trial in relapsed/transformed FL (and SLL) setting showed 30% CR (vs. 16% with rituximab) and 14-month median duration of response (vs. 12 months) after a median of two prior treatments.[42]
  - Dose is 0.4 mCi/kg or 0.3 mCi/kg for patients with mild thrombocytopenia (platelets 100,000 to 150,000/μL).
  - Proportion of patients with durable CR identified, with median response duration of 28 months.
  - Chemotherapy and ASCT tolerated well post-Zevalin.
- Bexxar: in relapsed/transformed setting
  - Dose: individualized to give 75 cGy of TBI
  - Twenty percent CR, 6.5-month median duration of response after a median of four treatments in a pivotal trial of 60 chemotherapy-refractory rituximab-naïve patients with low-grade and transformed lymphomas.[43]
  - Thirty-two percent had durable responses of 1 year or more, with median duration of 46 months.[44]
  - MDS/AML was seen, but occurred in patients with prior chemotherapy.[45]
  - Untreated FL: 75% CR, of which 80% is PCR negative, 5-year PFS 59% in 76 patients.[46]
    - The study was criticized for treating some patients who had low tumor burden and would ordinarily be observed.
    - No MDS/AML after 5.1-year median follow-up, bolstering safety.
- Chemo-radioimmunotherapy: phase II studies
  - CHOP–Bexxar: CR/CRu increased from 39% after CHOP to 69% after Bexxar, with 5-year OS of 87% and PFS of 67% in untreated patients.[47]
  - Phase III CHOP–Bexxar vs. R-CHOP study ongoing
- RIT offers the ease of one treatment and a possibility of long-term remission in a small number of patients; the drawback is price and the need to use radionuclides in collaboration with nuclear medicine or radiation oncology physicians.

- Vaccines
  - Of all lymphomas, FL has the most evidence for vaccine efficacy.
  - Usual strategy is to vaccinate people to idiotype (Id, a unique antigen from the variable region composed of parts of immunoglobulin heavy and light chains that are expressed by a malignant clone) coupled to immunogenic carrier (KLH, keyhole limpet hemocyanin) with a goal of eliciting both T-cell and anti-Id antibody responses.
    - To increase immunogenicity, dendritic cells can be exposed to vaccine ex vivo and reinfused or vaccine can be co-administered with GM-CSF.
  - A landmark trial of an idiotype-specific vaccine was conducted at Stanford with 40 FL patients given standard chemotherapy.
    - Twenty patients demonstrating immune response had increased freedom from progression (FFP) (7.9 vs. 1.3 years) and median OS (not reached vs. 7 years).[48]
  - Bendandi et al.[49] administered Id vaccine with GM-CSF to 20 patients in first CR.
    - Eight of 11 patients with detectable t(14;18) entered and maintained molecular CR, with 18 of 20 patients in CR at median follow-up of 42 months.
  - Timmerman et al.[50] infused dendritic cells pulsed with Id vaccine into 35 patients.
    - Sixteen of 23 patients who completed vaccination in first remission maintained remission at median of 43 months.
  - Three large phase III trials have recently completed accrual, results pending.
    - Phase II trial of four weekly rituximab doses followed (in patients with responding or stable disease) by immunization schedule with individualized Id-KLH vaccine (FavId) reported improvement in ORR from 47% to 63%, with median time to best response of 9 months from rituximab initiation, with such late response suggesting that FavId may be responsible for this improvement.[51]

- Proteasome inhibitors:
  - Bortezomib is a boronic acid inhibitor of 26S protea-some complex.
  - In FL, this inhibition could lead to reduction of bcl-2 levels by preventing degradation of IκBκ repressor of NFkB.
  - In a phase II trial, bortezomib had ORR of 58%, CR 10% in FL, with durable remissions after a median of three prior treatments.[52]
- Autologous transplantation: remains controversial
  - Auto-transplantation generally has not been a desir-able option due to high toxicity in a setting of indo-lent disease course with frequent bone marrow contamination.
    - All major prospective trials of ASCT were con-ducted without anti-CD20 therapy.
  - ASCT was used in first CR/PR in three randomized trials with prolongation of PFS but only one demon-strated borderline OS improvement.
    - ASCT vs. IFN maintenance in first CR/PR demon-strated improved 5-year PFS (65% vs. 33%) in a German study of low-grade lymphoma.[53]
      - Increased rates of MDS/AML were seen with ASCT in this study, as well as several others, making ASCT less desirable.
    - ASCT vs. CHVP/IFN in first CR/PR did not show statistically significant improvement in 7-year event-free survival (38% vs. 28%, $P=.11$) or OS (76% vs. 71%, $P=0.53$) even though OS had bor-derline significance in a prior report.[54]
  - ASCT vs. chemotherapy in relapse: the CUP trial
    - Eighty-nine patients with relapsed/progressive FL in CR/PR after three cycles of CHOP went on to three cycles of CHOP or cytoxan/TBI followed by purged or unpurged stem cell rescue in preritux-imab era.[55]
    - Chemotherapy arm had lower OS at 4 years (46% vs. 71/77% unpurged/purged ASCT) without clear benefit of purging.

- The trial was criticized for closing prior to accrual goals, unplanned analysis, and clinical risk factor imbalance between groups.
- Use of rituximab and RIT as in vivo purging and of in vitro monoclonal antibody-based purging increases the frequency of PCR negative stem cell product.
  - PCR negativity correlates with longer remission in transplant as well as in nontransplant settings, as mentioned above.
  - Dana Farber experience showed that in 153 patients with in vitro purging between 1985 and 1995 (and only 30% CR at bone marrow harvest), 8-year post–ASCT DFS was 42% and OS was 66%, with 69% OS from diagnosis at 12 years.[56]
- ASCT remains experimental, with promising use of rituximab and RIT that could yield better outcomes with less MDS/AML.
- Allogeneic transplantation: the only modality known to cure
  - Graft versus lymphoma effect plays a significant role in FL, because donor lymphocyte infusions have converted a good proportion of patients to CR.
  - Allo-SCT results in lower relapse but is significantly more toxic than ASCT with treatment-related mortality (TRM) of 30%.
  - International Bone Marrow Transplant Registry compared 176 FL patients who underwent allo-SCT with 131 patients who had purged and 597 patients who had unpurged ASCT (Figure 3-3).[57]
    - Five-year TRM: 30%, 14%, 8%; recurrence: 21%, 43%, 58%; 5-year OS: 51%, 62%, 55%, respectively
    - No significant incidence of MDS/AML noted
  - Non-myeloablateive ("mini") allo-SCT may have lower TRM.
    - In a European Bone Marrow Transplant registry study of 188 patients, 52 with low-grade lymphoma, TRM was 12% at 100 days and 31% at 2 years, and 2-year OS was 65%.[58]
    - Morris et al.[59] treated 88 patients (41 with low-grade lymphomas) with alemtuzumab, melphalan,

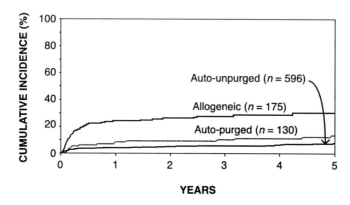

Figure 3-3: Cumulative incidences of treatment-related mortality by type of transplant. Used with permission from *Blood,* Journal of the American Society of Hematology. Van Besien, K., 2003, Vol. 102: 3521–3529.

and fludarabine conditioning prior to allogeneic transplantation, 65 from siblings.
- TRM at 2 years was only 11%, with projected 3-year OS of 73%.

General Treatment Approach

- Early disease (I/nonbulky II):
  - IFRT, or
  - Observation until treatment criteria are met
- Advanced disease (bulky II/III/IV):
  - Observation until treatment criteria are met
  - IFRT for symptomatic sites whether or not systemic therapy is needed
  - Human leukocyte antigen typing of siblings for patients younger than 60 years
  - When decision to treat is made:
    - Rituximab in patients with low tumor burden and significant comorbidity, or
    - R-CVP (preferred), or
    - R-CHOP (preferred, particularly if high tumor burden), or
    - R-fludarabine (caution with patients older than 70), or

- Clinical trial with a low-toxicity investigational agent
- Maintenance rituximab should be considered (favor van Oers' or Ghielmini's schedules)
- At relapse:
  - Observation or treatments as per above, or
  - Clinical trial
  - Radioimmunotherapy, or
  - R-FCM (may follow by maintenance rituximab), or
- Second relapse and beyond:
  - Observation or treatments as per above
  - Clinical trial
  - RIT
  - ASCT or allo-SCT may be considered.

■ References

1. Fisher RI, LeBlanc M, Press OW, Maloney DG, Unger JM, Miller TP. New treatment options have changed the survival of patients with follicular lymphoma. *J Clin Oncol.* 2005; 23(33):8447–8452.
2. Mann RB, Berard CW. Criteria for the cytologic subclassification of follicular lymphomas: a proposed alternative method. *Hematological Oncology.* 1983;1(2):187–192.
3. Martin AR, Weisenburger DD, Chan WC, et al. Prognostic value of cellular proliferation and histologic grade in follicular lymphoma. *Blood.* 1995;85(12):3671–3678.
4. Glas AM, Kersten MJ, Delahaye LJ, et al. Gene expression profiling in follicular lymphoma to assess clinical aggressiveness and to guide the choice of treatment. *Blood.* 2005; 105(1):301–307.
5. Dave SS, Wright G, Tan B, et al. Prediction of survival in follicular lymphoma based on molecular features of tumor-infiltrating immune cells. *N Engl J Med.* 2004;351(21): 2159–2169.
6. Ott G, Katzenberger T, Lohr A, et al. Cytomorphologic, immunohistochemical, and cytogenetic profiles of follicular lymphoma: Two types of follicular lymphoma grade 3. *Blood.* 2002;99(10):3806–3812.
7. Hans CP, Weisenburger DD, Vose JM, et al. A significant diffuse component predicts for inferior survival in grade 3 follicular lymphoma, but cytologic subtypes do not predict survival. *Blood.* 2003;101(6):2363–2367.

8. Solal-Celigny P, Roy P, Colombat P, et al. Follicular lymphoma international prognostic index. *Blood.* 2004;104(5):1258–1265.

9. Buske C, Hoster E, Dreyling M, Hasford J, Unterhalt M, Hiddemann W. The Follicular Lymphoma International Prognostic Index (FLIPI) separates high-risk from intermediate- or low-risk patients with advanced-stage follicular lymphoma treated front-line with rituximab and the combination of cyclophosphamide, doxorubicin, vincristine, and prednisone (R-CHOP) with respect to treatment outcome. *Blood.* 2006;108(5):1504–1508.

10. Gine E, Montoto S, Bosch F, et al. The Follicular Lymphoma International Prognostic Index (FLIPI) and the histological subtype are the most important factors to predict histological transformation in follicular lymphoma. *Ann Oncol.* 2006;17(10):1539–1545.

11. Advani R, Rosenberg SA, Horning SJ. Stage I and II follicular non-Hodgkin's lymphoma: long-term follow-up of no initial therapy. *J Clin Oncol.* 2004;22(8):1454–1459.

12. Seymour JF, Pro B, Fuller LM, et al. Long-term follow-up of a prospective study of combined modality therapy for stage I-II indolent non-Hodgkin's lymphoma. *J Clin Oncol.* 2003;21(11):2115–2122.

13. Johnson PW, Rohatiner AZ, Whelan JS, et al. Patterns of survival in patients with recurrent follicular lymphoma: a 20-year study from a single center. *J Clin Oncol.* 1995;13(1):140–147.

14. Horning SJ, Rosenberg SA. The natural history of initially untreated low-grade non-Hodgkin's lymphomas. *N Engl J Med.* 1984;311(23):1471–1475.

15. Ardeshna KM, Smith P, Norton A, et al. Long-term effect of a watch and wait policy versus immediate systemic treatment for asymptomatic advanced-stage non-Hodgkin lymphoma: a randomised controlled trial. *Lancet.* 2003;362(9383):516–522.

16. Young RC, Longo DL, Glatstein E, Ihde DC, Jaffe ES, DeVita VT, Jr. The treatment of indolent lymphomas: watchful waiting v aggressive combined modality treatment. *Seminars in Hematology.* 1988;25(2 Suppl 2):11–16.

17. Brice P, Bastion Y, Lepage E, et al. Comparison in low-tumor-burden follicular lymphomas between an initial no-treatment policy, prednimustine, or interferon alfa: a

randomized study from the Groupe d'Etude des Lymphomes Folliculaires. Groupe d'Etude des Lymphomes de l'Adulte. *J Clin Oncol.* 1997;15(3):1110–1117.

18. Travis LB, Weeks J, Curtis RE, et al. Leukemia following low-dose total body irradiation and chemotherapy for non-Hodgkin's lymphoma. *J Clin Oncol.* 1996;14(2):565–571.

19. Peterson BA, Petroni GR, Frizzera G, et al. Prolonged single-agent versus combination chemotherapy in indolent follicular lymphomas: a study of the cancer and leukemia group B. *J Clin Oncol.* 2003;21(1):5–15.

20. Hagenbeek A, Eghbali H, Monfardini S, et al. Phase III intergroup study of fludarabine phosphate compared with cyclophosphamide, vincristine, and prednisone chemotherapy in newly diagnosed patients with stage III and IV low-grade malignant Non-Hodgkin's lymphoma. *J Clin Oncol.* 2006; 24(10):1590–1596.

21. Klasa RJ, Meyer RM, Shustik C, et al. Randomized phase III study of fludarabine phosphate versus cyclophosphamide, vincristine, and prednisone in patients with recurrent low-grade non-Hodgkin's lymphoma previously treated with an alkylating agent or alkylator-containing regimen. *J Clin Oncol.* 2002;20(24):4649–4654.

22. Kay AC, Saven A, Carrera CJ, et al. 2-Chlorodeoxyadenosine treatment of low-grade lymphomas. *J Clin Oncol.* 1992;10(3):371–377.

23. Flinn IW, Byrd JC, Morrison C, et al. Fludarabine and cyclophosphamide with filgrastim support in patients with previously untreated indolent lymphoid malignancies. *Blood.* 2000;96(1):71–75.

24. Velasquez WS, Lew D, Grogan TM, et al. Combination of fludarabine and mitoxantrone in untreated stages III and IV low-grade lymphoma: S9501. *J Clin Oncol.* 2003;21(10): 1996–2003.

25. McLaughlin P, Hagemeister FB, Romaguera JE, et al. Fludarabine, mitoxantrone, and dexamethasone: an effective new regimen for indolent lymphoma. *J Clin Oncol.* 1996;14(4):1262–1268.

26. Fisher RI, Dana BW, LeBlanc M, et al. Interferon alpha consolidation after intensive chemotherapy does not prolong the progression-free survival of patients with low-grade non-Hodgkin's lymphoma: results of the Southwest Oncology Group randomized phase III study 8809. *J Clin Oncol.* 2000;18(10):2010–2016.

27. Rohatiner AZ, Gregory WM, Peterson B, et al. Meta-analysis to evaluate the role of interferon in follicular lymphoma. *J Clin Oncol.* 2005;23(10):2215–2223.

28. McLaughlin P, Grillo-Lopez AJ, Link BK, et al. Rituximab chimeric anti-CD20 monoclonal antibody therapy for relapsed indolent lymphoma: half of patients respond to a four-dose treatment program. *J Clin Oncol.* 1998;16(8): 2825–2833.

29. Hainsworth JD, Burris HA, 3rd, Morrissey LH, et al. Rituximab monoclonal antibody as initial systemic therapy for patients with low-grade non-Hodgkin lymphoma. *Blood.* 2000;95(10):3052–3056.

30. Davis TA, Grillo-Lopez AJ, White CA, et al. Rituximab anti-CD20 monoclonal antibody therapy in non-Hodgkin's lymphoma: safety and efficacy of re-treatment. *J Clin Oncol.* 2000;18(17):3135–3143.

31. Ghielmini M, Schmitz SF, Cogliatti SB, et al. Prolonged treatment with rituximab in patients with follicular lymphoma significantly increases event-free survival and response duration compared with the standard weekly x 4 schedule. *Blood.* 2004;103(12):4416–4423.

32. Hainsworth JD, Litchy S, Shaffer DW, Lackey VL, Grimaldi M, Greco FA. Maximizing therapeutic benefit of rituximab: maintenance therapy versus re-treatment at progression in patients with indolent non-Hodgkin's lymphoma—a randomized phase II trial of the Minnie Pearl Cancer Research Network. *J Clin Oncol.* 2005;23(6):1088–1095.

33. Hochster HS, Weller E, Gascoyne RD, et al. Maintenance Rituximab after CVP Results in Superior Clinical Outcome in Advanced Follicular Lymphoma (FL): Results of the E1496 Phase III Trial from the Eastern Cooperative Oncology Group and the Cancer and Leukemia Group B. *Blood.* 2005;106(11):349a.

34. van Oers MH, Klasa R, Marcus RE, et al. Rituximab maintenance improves clinical outcome of relapsed/resistant follicular non-Hodgkin lymphoma in patients both with and without rituximab during induction: results of a prospective randomized phase 3 intergroup trial. *Blood.* 2006;108(10): 3295–3301.

35. Berinstein NL, Grillo-Lopez AJ, White CA, et al. Association of serum Rituximab (IDEC-C2B8) concentration and anti-tumor response in the treatment of recurrent low-grade or follicular non-Hodgkin's lymphoma. *Ann Oncol.* 1998;9(9):995–1001.

35. Gordan LN, Grow WB, Pusateri A, Douglas V, Mendenhall NP, Lynch JW. Phase II trial of individualized rituximab dosing for patients with CD20-positive lymphoproliferative disorders. *J Clin Oncol.* 2005;23(6):1096–1102.

37. Hiddemann W, Kneba M, Dreyling M, et al. Frontline therapy with rituximab added to the combination of cyclophosphamide, doxorubicin, vincristine, and prednisone (CHOP) significantly improves the outcome for patients with advanced-stage follicular lymphoma compared with therapy with CHOP alone: results of a prospective randomized study of the German Low-Grade Lymphoma Study Group. *Blood.* 2005;106(12):3725–3732.

38. Marcus R, Imrie K, Belch A, et al. CVP chemotherapy plus rituximab compared with CVP as first-line treatment for advanced follicular lymphoma. *Blood.* 2005;105(4): 1417–1423.

39. Forstpointner R, Dreyling M, Repp R, et al. The addition of rituximab to a combination of fludarabine, cyclophosphamide, mitoxantrone (FCM) significantly increases the response rate and prolongs survival as compared with FCM alone in patients with relapsed and refractory follicular and mantle cell lymphomas: results of a prospective randomized study of the German Low-Grade Lymphoma Study Group. *Blood.* 2004;104(10):3064–3071.

40. Forstpointner R, Unterhalt M, Dreyling M, et al. Maintenance therapy with rituximab leads to a significant prolongation of response duration after salvage therapy with a combination of rituximab, fludarabine, cyclophosphamide, and mitoxantrone (R-FCM) in patients with recurring and refractory follicular and mantle cell lymphomas: Results of a prospective randomized study of the German Low Grade Lymphoma Study Group (GLSG). *Blood.* 2006;108(13): 4003–4008.

41. Rambaldi A, Carlotti E, Oldani E, et al. Quantitative PCR of bone marrow BCL2/IgH+ cells at diagnosis predicts treatment response and long-term outcome in follicular non-Hodgkin lymphoma. *Blood.* 2005;105(9):3428–3433.

42. Witzig TE, Flinn IW, Gordon LI, et al. Treatment with ibritumomab tiuxetan radioimmunotherapy in patients with rituximab-refractory follicular non-Hodgkin's lymphoma. *J Clin Oncol.* 2002;20(15):3262–3269.

43. Kaminski MS, Zelenetz AD, Press OW, et al. Pivotal study of iodine I 131 tositumomab for chemotherapy-refractory

low-grade or transformed low-grade B-cell non-Hodgkin's lymphomas. *J Clin Oncol.* 2001;19(19):3918–3928.

44. Fisher RI, Kaminski MS, Wahl RL, et al. Tositumomab and iodine-131 tositumomab produces durable complete remissions in a subset of heavily pretreated patients with low-grade and transformed non-Hodgkin's lymphomas. *J Clin Oncol.* 2005;23(30):7565–7573.

45. Bennett JM, Kaminski MS, Leonard JP, et al. Assessment of treatment-related myelodysplastic syndromes and acute myeloid leukemia in patients with non-Hodgkin lymphoma treated with tositumomab and iodine I131 tositumomab. *Blood.* 2005;105(12):4576–4582.

46. Kaminski MS, Tuck M, Estes J, et al. 131I-tositumomab therapy as initial treatment for follicular lymphoma. *N Engl J Med.* 2005;352(5):441–449.

47. Press OW, Unger JM, Braziel RM, et al. Phase II trial of CHOP chemotherapy followed by tositumomab/iodine I-131 tositumomab for previously untreated follicular non-Hodgkin's lymphoma: five-year follow-up of Southwest Oncology Group Protocol S9911. *J Clin Oncol.* 2006; 24(25):4143–4149.

48. Hsu FJ, Caspar CB, Czerwinski D, et al. Tumor-specific idiotype vaccines in the treatment of patients with B-cell lymphoma—long-term results of a clinical trial. *Blood.* 1997; 89(9):3129–3135.

49. Bendandi M, Gocke CD, Kobrin CB, et al. Complete molecular remissions induced by patient-specific vaccination plus granulocyte-monocyte colony-stimulating factor against lymphoma. *Nat Med.* 1999;5(10):1171–1177.

50. Timmerman JM, Czerwinski DK, Davis TA, et al. Idiotype-pulsed dendritic cell vaccination for B-cell lymphoma: clinical and immune responses in 35 patients. *Blood.* 2002; 99(5):1517–1526.

51. Koc ON, Redfern C, Wiernik PH, et al. Active Immunotherapy with FavId® (Id/KLH) Following Rituximab Induction: Long-Term Follow-Up of Response Rate Improvement (RRI) and Disease Progression in Follicular Lymphoma Patients (pts). *Blood.* 2006;108(11): 691a.

52. O'Connor OA, Wright J, Moskowitz C, et al. Phase II clinical experience with the novel proteasome inhibitor bortezomib in patients with indolent non-Hodgkin's lymphoma and mantle cell lymphoma. *J Clin Oncol.* 2005;23(4):676–684.

53. Lenz G, Dreyling M, Schiegnitz E, et al. Myeloablative radiochemotherapy followed by autologous stem cell transplantation in first remission prolongs progression-free survival in follicular lymphoma: results of a prospective, randomized trial of the German Low-Grade Lymphoma Study Group. *Blood*. 2004;104(9):2667–2674.

54. Sebban C, Mounier N, Brousse N, et al. Standard chemotherapy with interferon compared with CHOP followed by high-dose therapy with autologous stem cell transplantation in untreated patients with advanced follicular lymphoma: the GELF-94 randomized study from the Groupe d'Etude des Lymphomes de l'Adulte (GELA). *Blood*. 2006;108(8):2540–2544.

52. Schouten HC, Qian W, Kvaloy S, et al. High-dose therapy improves progression-free survival and survival in relapsed follicular non-Hodgkin's lymphoma: results from the randomized European CUP trial. *J Clin Oncol*. 2003;21(21): 3918–3927.

53. Freedman AS, Neuberg D, Mauch P, et al. Long-term follow-up of autologous bone marrow transplantation in patients with relapsed follicular lymphoma. *Blood*. 1999; 94(10):3325–3333.

55. van Besien K, Loberiza FR, Jr., Bajorunaite R, et al. Comparison of autologous and allogeneic hematopoietic stem cell transplantation for follicular lymphoma. *Blood*. 2003;102(10):3521–3529.

56. Robinson SP, Goldstone AH, Mackinnon S, et al. Chemoresistant or aggressive lymphoma predicts for a poor outcome following reduced-intensity allogeneic progenitor cell transplantation: an analysis from the Lymphoma Working Party of the European Group for Blood and Bone Marrow Transplantation. *Blood*. 2002;100(13):4310–4316.

59. Morris E, Thomson K, Craddock C, et al. Outcomes after alemtuzumab-containing reduced-intensity allogeneic transplantation regimen for relapsed and refractory non-Hodgkin lymphoma. *Blood*. 2004;104(13):3865–3871.

CHAPTER 4

Marginal Zone Lymphoma

■ Three Distinct Clinical Entities

* Extranodal marginal zone B-cell lymphoma (MZL) of mucosa-associated lymphoid tissue (MALT) most common of the three types
* Nodal marginal zone lymphoma
* Splenic marginal zone lymphoma (with or without villous lymphocytes)

■ Extranodal MZL of MALT

Epidemiology

* Five percent of non-Hodgkin's lymphoma (NHL), 40% of gastric lymphomas
* Indolent, usually localized B-cell lymphoma with associated antigen-driven proliferation and excellent survival
* Involves epithelial gland surfaces, with stomach being the most common site
* Other MALT sites could be involved: lung (also known as bronchial associated lymphoid tissue), breast, thyroid, orbit, conjunctiva, oral cavity, skin, and lacrimal and salivary glands.
* Average age of presentation is 60 years with wide distribution, slight female predominance.
* Several infections and autoimmune disorders are thought to contribute to persistent immune up-regulation that eventually becomes antigen independent.
    * Gastric MZL: *H. pylori*–caused chronic gastritis is the best-documented association, with evidence of *H. pylori* antigens causing immune proliferation; regression of early lesions with antibiotic therapy for *H. pylori*.
    * Other associated diseases and sites of involvement:
        * Sjogren's syndrome (4–7% of patients)—salivary and lacrimal ducts

- Hashimoto's thyroiditis (0.5–1.5% of patients)—thyroid
- *Borrelia afzelii* infection (European Lyme disease)—cutaneous lymphoma and lymphocytoma
- *Chlamydia psittaci*—ocular adnexal lymphoma (the strength of association varies widely between studies)

Presentation

- Site-dependent complaints (i.e., heartburn, sicca syndrome), often with antecedent or concurrent diagnosis of above infectious or autoimmune disorder.
- MZL presenting at nongastric extranodal sites may involve the stomach upon testing in up to a third of patients.[1]
  - Gastrointestinal (GI) evaluation, including *H. pylori* testing, should be considered in non-GI presentation.
- Usually localized, with 30–35% with stage III/IV disease
  - Gastric MZL is usually localized, whereas nongastric MZL has increased frequency of disseminated disease and of spread to other MALT sites.
- B symptoms up to 20%, bone marrow (BM) involvement up to 15%
- Monoclonal gammopathy in up to a third of patients, implying plasmacytoid differentiation
- May transform to diffuse large B-cell lymphoma (DLBCL); 70% of DLBCL at MALT sites is found with MZL component, with DLBCL presumed to originate from MZL transformation
- Fluorine-18 fluoro-deoxyglucose positron emission tomography scanning is less sensitive in MZL than in follicular lymphoma.

Pathology

Morphology

- Resembles normal marginal zones of lymphoid tissue
- Heterogenous-appearing small B lymphocytes, with marginal zone centrocyte-like cells, monocytoid cells, and plasma cells, few or no large lymphocytes

- Located in the marginal or interfollicular zones with reactive follicles
- Presence of clusters or sheets of large cells suggests transformation to DBLCL, although some investigators call it "high-grade MALT lymphoma."

Immunophenotype

- B-cell antigens (CD 19, 20, 22, 79a); monoclonal surface immunoglobulins (predominantly IgM as in follicular lymphoma), but not IgD; complement receptors (CD21, CD35).
- Forty to 60% have monoclonal cytoplasmic Ig (plasmacytoid differentiation).
- CD5 negative, CD10 negative, CD23 negative
- Normal cyclin D1 and bcl-2

Cytogenetic and Molecular Changes

- Immunoglobulin genes rearranged, with somatic hypermutation, indicating postgerminal cell origin
- Ig variable regions similar to those in autoantibodies and rheumatoid factor
- Trisomy 3 (60%) and t(11;18) (25–40%) are mutually exclusive abnormalities.
    - t(11;18): API2/MALT1 fusion, with API2 (apoptosis-inhibitor 2) likely inhibiting apoptosis, and MALT1, which is thought to be important in NFκB signaling
    - t(11;18)–positive disease is usually more advanced, *H. pylori* independent, has no other cytogenetic abnormalities, and is less likely to transform.
    - Trisomy 3–positive disease is less advanced, initially *H. pylori* dependent, contains additional cytogenetic abnormalities, and is more likely to transform.
- Other abnormalities:
    - t(14;18) with IgH/MALT1 translocation occurs in up to 15–20% of MZL cases, usually nongastric ones, which results in MALT1 deregulation.
    - t(1;14)—BCL10/IgH translocation, seen in 1–2% of MZL including gastric cases, results in overexpression of BCL10.

- ■ It often is resistant to *H. pylori* therapy.
  - • Translocations involving FOXP1 and BCL-6 genes may rarely be involved.
- ■ The common pathway of molecular abnormalities seems to be coupling of BCL10 and MALT1 signals, resulting in constitutive NFκB pathway activation.

Prognosis

- ■ Overall, high complete remission (CR) rates and long-term survival (80% at 10 years).
- ■ Monoclonal gammopathy relates to plasmacytoid differentiation and more advanced disease.
- ■ Advanced stage (disseminated disease) may not affect prognosis in nongastric MZL, while it likely does for gastric MZL.
  - • German series of 371 patients with GI lymphomas showed that small bowel or multiple GI sites have worse overall survival (OS) than gastric and ileocecal lymphomas; higher-stage disease had worse OS, but higher grade (i.e., DLBCL) had similar OS but worse event-free survival (EFS).[2]
  - • Whereas a review of 180 patients with nongastric MZL of MALT showed that higher stage was associated with worse OS, nodal involvement with lower cause-specific survival, and International Prognostic Index (IPI) greater than 2 with worse progression-free survival.[3] Another review of 158 patients specifically looked at disseminated disease and noted no difference in survival.[1]
- ■ Depth of invasion, t(11;18), nuclear expression of bcl-10, and NFκB correlates with *H. pylori* independence.
- ■ If MZL found with DLBCL in GI tract, prognosis is likely better than with DLBCL alone.

Treatment

- ■ Early disease (I/II):
  - • If *H. pylori* positive, start with antibiotic therapy.
    - ■ Several triple-therapy regimens eradicate *H. pylori* in more than 90% of patients: proton pump inhibitor twice a day (bid), amoxicillin 1g bid (or

metronidazole 500 bid if penicillin-allergic), and clarithromycin 500 mg bid for 2 weeks.

- CR was 62% in 90 patients with stage IE disease, with 4 or 56 of those in CR relapsing with median follow-up of 45 months.[4]
- Similarly, 55% histologic CR was seen in 189 patients with stage I disease.
  - However, only 44% of those tested remained in molecular remission by polymerase chain reaction (PCR) (for rearranged IgH) at median of 2 years after treatment, without a correlation with histological relapse.[5]
  - This corroborated an earlier German study with 45% of patients remaining PCR positive at median of 20.5 months after achieving CR; 4 of those 20 patients relapsed.[6]
- It is thus unclear if antibiotic therapy results in cures; longer follow-up is needed.
- Antibiotics probably work best for mucosal (i.e., shallow) stage IE disease, which constitutes only about 10% of all gastric lymphomas.
- If *H. pylori* negative, treat with radiation therapy (30 Gy) or surgical resection (more morbid).
  - Initial report of 30 Gy radiation therapy (RT) in 17 patients with stage I/II disease negative for or resistant to *H. pylori* demonstrated EFS of 100% at median follow-up of 27 months.[7]
  - Retrospective review of 93 patients with IE/IIE disease treated with median 30 Gy of involved field radiation therapy (IFRT) (8 with chemotherapy) showed 5-year disease-free survival (DFS) of 77% and OS of 98%.
    - No relapses were seen in gastric or thyroid MZL, whereas other sites relapsed contralaterally or distantly in 22%.[8]
- If still *H. pylori* positive on recheck endoscopy at 3–6 months after treatment, treat again before moving to RT or resection.

- *H. pylori* treatment also works for small intestine and rectum sites, but would not be expected to work for most other nongastric MZL.
- Still refractory or relapsed: rituximab
  - Twenty-seven refractory to prior therapy (mostly antibiotics based), 4 with stage IV: CR 46%, only 2 relapses at median follow-up of 33 months.[9]
- Advanced (III/IV) or multiple relapsed disease: treatment is similar to that in FL but response is probably better due to lower tumor burden.
  - Rituximab: a study of 35 patients, 20 with stage IV, showed 43% CR, median duration of response 10.5 months, both higher in chemotherapy-naïve patients.[10]
  - Single-agent alkylators: oral daily chlorambucil or cyclophosphamide for 12–24 months yielded 75% CR in 24 patients (7 with stage IV disease), with about 50% still in CR at mean follow-up of 45 months.[11]
    - Chlorambucil induced 55% CR in *H. pylori* treatment nonresponders, higher if no lymph nodes were seen on endoscopic ultrasound.[12]
  - Purine analogs: cladribine had 84% CR in a study of 26 patients, 3 patients who did not achieve CR had nongastric MZL.[13]
  - In a German study, four cycles of CVP were successfully used prior to RT in 34 patients with stage IIE disease with over 90% 5-year OS.[14]
  - FM vs. CVP: in nongastric stage IE MZL, both regimens achieved CR, but 4 of 11 patients treated with CVP relapsed and were salvaged by FM.[15]
  - Overall, with the combination of chemotherapy and RT for local control, 5-year OS is over 90% for all of the options above.
- Transformation:
  - Cyclophosphamide, doxorubicin, and prednisone (CHOP)–based therapy should be used without delay, particularly with higher stage disease and isolated DLCBL without MZL component.
  - Reports have been made of antibiotic response of *H. pylori*–positive "high-grade MALT lymphoma."

- Fifteen of 16 patients with stage IE disease had *H. pylori* eradicated and 10 (63%) had CR maintained at median follow-up of 43 months; remaining 5 of 6 patients had CR after CHOP.[16]
- Unlike with antibiotic therapy, 70% of *H. pylori*–positive lymphomas (16 of 20 containing DLBCL) treated with CHOP and RT became PCR negative.[17]

■ Variants

Alpha-Chain Disease

- Also known as immunoproliferative small intestine disease or Mediterranean lymphoma
- Affects young adults, mean age 25–30 years, equal gender distribution, Middle East/Africa, low socioeconomic status
- Presents with intermittent abdominal pain and diarrhea and malabsorption
- Often relapses and presents with transformation to DLBCL or Burkitt's lymphoma
- Proximal intestine thickening, nodularity, or erythema on esophagogastroduodenoscopy
- Mucosa infiltrated by small centrocyte-like lymphocytes and plasma cells (centroblasts or immunoblasts if transformed)
- Produces truncated alpha-heavy chains (hence the name), detected in serum
- Associated with *Campylobacter jejuni* infection[18]
- Early stage disease responds to antibiotic treatment, with 30–70% CR; advanced/transformed disease is given CHOP-like regimens.[19]

Splenic MZL

Epidemiology

- Less than 5% of NHL, 1–2% of CLL on BM, up to 25% of indolent B-cell lymphomas/leukemias in splenectomies
- A diagnosis of exclusion with chronic B-cell leukemia and on splenectomy

- Splenic MZL with villous lymphocytes is associated with hepatitis C infection.
- Middle aged to older adults, median age 65, no gender predilection

Presentation

- Almost always presents with splenomegaly and lymphocytosis
- Ninety percent present with stage IV disease: peripheral blood, BM, and liver.
- Up to 40% have hepatomegaly, rarely lymphadenopathy.
- Monoclonal gammopathy present in up to a third (again, IgM).
- Autoimmune events present in up to a fifth.

Pathology

Morphology

- Splenic white pulp: central residual germinal centers are surrounded by expanded mantle and marginal zones that are involved by lymphoma.
  - Neoplastic cells in the mantle zone are small, with slight nuclear irregularity, little cytoplasm.
  - Those in the marginal zone are larger, with more dispersed chromatin and more abundant pale cytoplasm, with larger cells present.
- Splenic red pulp: infiltrated in nodular and diffuse patterns, with frequent sinus infiltration and presence of epithelioid histiocytes.
- Splenic hilar lymph nodes: often involved by vaguely nodular infiltrate.
- BM: nodular interstitial involvement.
- Peripheral blood: abundant cytoplasm, plasmacytoid or with surface "villous" projections.

Immunophenotype

- B-cell antigens (CD19, CD20, CD22), surface IgM and IgD positive, bcl-2 positive
- CD5 negative, CD10 negative, CD23 negative, CD43 negative

* Express adhesion receptors CD29, CD44, CD49d, LFA-1, and ICAM-1
* Differs from the other B-cell neoplasm with cellular projections, hairy cell leukemia, in that it does not express CD25 or CD103.

Cytogenetic and Molecular Changes

* Somatic hypermutation seen in at least half the cases; may be subject to antigen selection.
* Deletions 7q21–32 (up to 40%); trisomy 3 less common (17–35%), but not t(11;18), as in extranodal MZL.
* p53 abnormalities in 17%
* In one gene-expression profile (GEP), genes associated with intracellular signaling via the AKT1 pathway were up-regulated.[20]
* A GEP of 44 patients that was correlated with tissue microarray demonstrated up-regulation of B-cell receptor, tumor necrosis factor signaling, and NFκB activation genes.[21]

Prognosis

* Survival 72–90% at 5 years; median survival 9–13 years
* No survival difference based on presence of villous lymphocytes.
* Anemia and lymphocytosis over 16×10^9 per L were risk factors, and splenectomy was beneficial in one study of 129 patients,[22] while a recent review of 309 patients confirmed adverse prognostic significance of anemia, defined as hemoglobin less than 12, as well as of elevated lactate dehydrogenase (LDH), and of albumin less than 3.5 g/dL. [23]
* Unmutated IgV, 7q interstitial deletions, p53 abnormalities prognostically worse
* CD38 positivity, unmutated IgVh, and expression of NFκB pathway genes predicted shorter survival in the GEP of 44 patients mentioned above, and all had down-regulation of 7q genes.

Treatment

* Observe first, as with other indolent lymphomas.
* If treatment is needed, usually due to cytopenias or symptomatic splenomegaly, consider splenectomy first,

because it can cause long-term remissions, the majority of them partial.[24]

■ Rituximab with alkylators or purine analogs, with or without splenectomy, is effective.

• Note that splenic MZL may be more resistant to chemotherapy than FL or small lymphatic lymphoma/chronic lymphocytic leukemia.

■ Single-agent rituximab caused responses in 10 of 11 patients, with 8 having resolution of splenomegaly and cytopenias and no evidence of progression at median 21-month follow-up.[25]

■ Retrospective review of 70 patients from MD Anderson showed better failure-free and overall survival with rituximab as a single agent or in combination with purine-analog-based chemotherapy than with chemotherapy alone.[26]

• Single agent rituximab resulted in resolution of splenomegaly in 92% of the patients, with better count normalization as compared to those undergoing splenectomy.

• Single agent rituximab may become a viable alternative to splenectomy.

■ Splenic MZL with villous lymphocytes: if hepatitis C virus (HCV) positive, treat HCV (currently with interferon [IFN], with or without ribavirin); those that clear HCV RNA have prolonged remissions.[27]

Nodal MZL

■ MZL that appears exclusively in lymph nodes
■ A diagnosis of exclusion after extranodal MZL, splenic MZL, and other lymphomas have been ruled out
■ Rare—1% of NHL, median age of onset about 50 years, slight female predominance
■ Presents with asymptomatic lymphadenopathy, BM involvement in 32–43%, advanced stage in 70%
■ Morphology appears similar to either extranodal MZL (monocytoid, preserved mantle zones and germinal centers) or to splenic MZL (marginal zone cell infiltrates with smaller mantle zones).

- If monocytoid differentiation—if has Sjogren's, it is likely extranodal MZL.
- Immunophenotype is same as extranodal MZL (CD5 negative, CD10 negative, CD23 negative, IgD negative) or splenic MZL (IgD positive).
- Due to rarity and biphenotypic definition, prognosis and treatment are difficult to define.
  - Nodal MZL more commonly presents with advanced disease, peripheral and para-aortic lymphadenopathy, less commonly presents with a mass greater than 5 cm, and has lower FFS and OS (56% vs. 81% at 5 years) than extranodal MZL of MALT even if only patients with IPI scores 0 to 3 are considered.[28]
  - A retrospective review of 124 patients with non–MALT MZL included 37 patients with nodal MZL. There was quick progression despite the use of CHOP-like and high-dose therapy, with median survival of 5.5 years, more similar to aggressive lymphomas.[29]
- Treatment: Nodal MZL is probably more aggressive than average indolent lymphomas. Multiagent chemotherapy with anthracycline, with or without rituximab, with or without RT, should be considered front line.

■ General Treatment Approach

Extranodal MZL

- Early stage (I/II):
  - If *H. pylori*–positive gastric MZL, antibiotic therapy
    - Recheck in 3–6 months, if still positive re-treat with antibiotics.
      - If *H. pylori*–negative or nongastric MZL: 30 Gy IFRT
- Advanced stage (III/IV) or relapsed (after antibiotic and IFRT failure):
  - Observe until treatment criteria are met
  - Rituximab, or purine analog (fludarabine or cladribine), or alkylator (cyclophosphamide or chlorambucil)
  - May consider combination therapy with agents above, or FM, or CVP

Splenic MZL

- Observe until treatment criteria are met.
- If decided to treat:
  - Splenectomy
  - If splenectomy contraindicated, consider splenic irradiation, single-agent rituximab, or chemoimmunotherapy, as with relapse.
  - If relapses, rituximab with purine analog (fludarabine) or/and alkylator (cyclophosphamide or chlorambucil).
  - If with villous lymphocytes and HCV, IFN alpha and ribavirin

Nodal MZL (Rare)

- Treat more similarly to aggressive than to indolent lymphomas.
- Consider starting with R-CHOP with or without IFRT.

■ References

1. Thieblemont C, Berger F, Dumontet C, et al. Mucosa-associated lymphoid tissue lymphoma is a disseminated disease in one third of 158 patients analyzed. *Blood.* 2000; 95(3):802–806.

2. Koch P, del Valle F, Berdel WE, et al. Primary gastrointestinal non-Hodgkin's lymphoma: I. Anatomic and histologic distribution, clinical features, and survival data of 371 patients registered in the German Multicenter Study GIT NHL 01/92. *J Clin Oncol.* 2001;19(18):3861–3873.

3. Zucca E, Conconi A, Pedrinis E, et al. Nongastric marginal zone B-cell lymphoma of mucosa-associated lymphoid tissue. *Blood.* 2003;101(7):2489–2495.

4. Fischbach W, Goebeler-Kolve ME, Dragosics B, Greiner A, Stolte M. Long-term outcome of patients with gastric marginal zone B cell lymphoma of mucosa associated lymphoid tissue (MALT) following exclusive *Helicobacter pylori* eradication therapy: experience from a large prospective series. *Gut.* 2004;53(1):34–37.

5. Bertoni F, Conconi A, Capella C, et al. Molecular follow-up in gastric mucosa-associated lymphoid tissue lymphomas: early analysis of the LY03 cooperative trial. *Blood.* 2002; 99(7):2541–2544.

6.   Thiede C, Wundisch T, Alpen B, et al. Long-term persistence of monoclonal B cells after cure of Helicobacter pylori infection and complete histologic remission in gastric mucosa-associated lymphoid tissue B-cell lymphoma. *J Clin Oncol.* 2001;19(6):1600–1609.

7.   Schechter NR, Portlock CS, Yahalom J. Treatment of mucosa-associated lymphoid tissue lymphoma of the stomach with radiation alone. *J Clin Oncol.* 1998;16(5):1916–1921.

8.   Tsang RW, Gospodarowicz MK, Pintilie M, et al. Localized mucosa-associated lymphoid tissue lymphoma treated with radiation therapy has excellent clinical outcome. *J Clin Oncol.* 2003;21(22):4157–4164.

9.   Martinelli G, Laszlo D, Ferreri AJ, et al. Clinical activity of rituximab in gastric marginal zone non-Hodgkin's lymphoma resistant to or not eligible for anti-Helicobacter pylori therapy. *J Clin Oncol.* 2005;23(9):1979–1983.

10.   Conconi A, Martinelli G, Thieblemont C, et al. Clinical activity of rituximab in extranodal marginal zone B-cell lymphoma of MALT type. *Blood.* 2003;102(8):2741–2745.

11.   Hammel P, Haioun C, Chaumette MT, et al. Efficacy of single-agent chemotherapy in low-grade B-cell mucosa-associated lymphoid tissue lymphoma with prominent gastric expression. *J Clin Oncol.* 1995;13(10):2524–2529.

12.   Levy M, Copie-Bergman C, Traulle C, et al. Conservative treatment of primary gastric low-grade B-cell lymphoma of mucosa-associated lymphoid tissue: predictive factors of response and outcome. *Am J Gastroenterol.* 2002;97(2): 292–297.

13.   Jager G, Neumeister P, Brezinschek R, et al. Treatment of extranodal marginal zone B-cell lymphoma of mucosa-associated lymphoid tissue type with cladribine: a phase II study. *J Clin Oncol.* 2002;20(18):3872–3877.

14.   Koch P, del Valle F, Berdel WE, et al. Primary gastrointestinal non-Hodgkin's lymphoma: II. Combined surgical and conservative or conservative management only in localized gastric lymphoma—results of the prospective German Multicenter Study GIT NHL 01/92. *J Clin Oncol.* 2001; 19(18):3874–3883.

15.   Zinzani PL, Stefoni V, Musuraca G, et al. Fludarabine-containing chemotherapy as frontline treatment of nongastrointestinal mucosa-associated lymphoid tissue lymphoma. *Cancer.* 2004;100(10):2190–2194.

16.   Chen LT, Lin JT, Shyu RY, et al. Prospective study of Helico-bacter pylori eradication therapy in stage I(E) high-grade

mucosa-associated lymphoid tissue lymphoma of the stomach. *J Clin Oncol.* 2001;19(22):4245–4251.

17. Alpen B, Kuse R, Parwaresch R, Muller-Hermelink HK, Stolte M, Neubauer A. Ongoing monoclonal B-cell proliferation is not common in gastric B-cell lymphoma after combined radiochemotherapy. *J Clin Oncol.* 2004;22(15): 3039–3045.

18. Lecuit M, Abachin E, Martin A, et al. Immunoproliferative small intestinal disease associated with *Campylobacter jejuni. N Engl J Med.* 2004;350(3):239–248.

19. Al-Saleem T, Al-Mondhiry H. Immunoproliferative small intestinal disease (IPSID): a model for mature B-cell neoplasms. *Blood.* 2005;105(6):2274–2280.

20. Thieblemont C, Nasser V, Felman P, et al. Small lymphocytic lymphoma, marginal zone B-cell lymphoma, and mantle cell lymphoma exhibit distinct gene-expression profiles allowing molecular diagnosis. *Blood.* 2004;103(7): 2727–2737.

21. Ruiz-Ballesteros E, Mollejo M, Rodriguez A, et al. Splenic marginal zone lymphoma: proposal of new diagnostic and prognostic markers identified after tissue and cDNA microarray analysis. *Blood.* 2005;106(5):1831–1838.

22. Parry-Jones N, Matutes E, Gruszka-Westwood AM, Swansbury GJ, Wotherspoon AC, Catovsky D. Prognostic features of splenic lymphoma with villous lymphocytes: a report on 129 patients. *Br J Haematol.* 2003;120(5):759–764.

23. Arcaini L, Lazzarino M, Colombo N, et al. Splenic marginal zone lymphoma: a prognostic model for clinical use. *Blood.* 2006;107(12):4643–4649.

24. Thieblemont C, Felman P, Callet-Bauchu E, et al. Splenic marginal-zone lymphoma: a distinct clinical and pathological entity. *The Lancet Oncology.* 2003;4(2):95–103.

25. Bennett Haematologica 2005. Bennett M, Sharma K, Yegena S, Gavish I, Dave HP, Schechter GP. Rituximab monotherapy for splenic marginal zone lymphoma. *Haematologica.* 2005;90(6):856–858.

26. Tsimberidou AM, Catovsky D, Schlette E, et al. Outcomes in patients with splenic marginal zone lymphoma and marginal zone lymphoma treated with rituximab with or without chemotherapy or chemotherapy alone. *Cancer.* 2006; 107(1):125–135.

27. Saadoun D, Suarez F, Lefrere F, et al. Splenic lymphoma with villous lymphocytes, associated with type II cryoglobulinemia and HCV infection: a new entity? *Blood.* 2005; 105(1):74–76.

28. Nathwani BN, Anderson JR, Armitage JO, et al. Marginal zone B-cell lymphoma: A clinical comparison of nodal and mucosa-associated lymphoid tissue types. Non-Hodgkin's Lymphoma Classification Project. *J Clin Oncol.* 1999; 17(8):2486–2492.
29. Berger F, Felman P, Thieblemont C, et al. Non-MALT marginal zone B-cell lymphomas: a description of clinical presentation and outcome in 124 patients. *Blood.* 2000;95(6): 1950–1956.

CHAPTER 5

Mantle Cell Lymphoma

■ Epidemiology

- Representing 5–7% of all non-Hodgkin's lymphomas (NHLs), mantle cell lymphoma (MCL) was identified as a separate subtype of NHL in 1992 and incorporated into the NHL classification in 1997.
- Median age of onset 60; male to female ratio 3:1
- Has worst features of both indolent and aggressive lymphomas: incurability and quick growth
- Chemo- and radiosensitive disease that tends to relapse, with average survival of 3–4 years that has not been changed by treatment
  - Southwestern Oncology Group retrospective review reported 10-year overall survival (OS) of 8%.[1]
  - Historically thought of as indolent, but due to its clinical course is now usually classified as aggressive lymphoma
- Rare cases may occur as part of familial lymphoproliferative disease, with anticipation effect.

■ Presentation

- B symptoms in about 30%
- Site-specific complaints, including increasing but painless lymphadenopathy and gastrointestinal (GI) and genitourinary symptoms (including those due to obstruction).
- About 55% present with intermediate risk International Prognostic Index (IPI) of 2 to 3, the rest split evenly between low-risk and high-risk groups.
- Advanced stage in 80–90%, with multiple organ involvement:
  - Nodal (80%): lymph nodes (70%), spleen (50%), Waldeyer's ring

* Extranodal (80%): bone marrow (BM) greater than 60%, GI tract 30% (lymphomatoid polyposis on colonoscopy), peripheral blood 30% (more if flow cytometry is performed)
    * Less commonly involved organs include parotids, skin, lung, and breast.
* Routine staging should included BM biopsy; if there are GI complaints, colonoscopy should be performed.

■ Pathology

Morphology

* Monotonous small to medium-sized lymphocytes with irregular nuclear borders and condensed chromatin without distinct nucleoli.
    * May mimic small lymphatic lymphoma/chronic lymphocytic leukemia with smaller round lymphocytes containing condensed chromatin or marginal zone B-cell lymphoma with abundant pale cytoplasm.
* Two blastoid variants:
    * Classic: lymphoblast-like with dispersed chromatin and high mitotic index
    * Pleiomorphic: heterogeneous lymphocytes with large cleaved nuclei and sometimes prominent nucleoli
* Lymph nodes have three patterns of involvement: mantle zone, nodular, or diffuse.
    * Mantle zone pattern: neoplastic cells expand only the mantle zones.
    * Nodular pattern: no normal germinal centers, neoplastic cells form vague follicle-like nodules.
    * Diffuse pattern: loss of any resemblance to normal architecture
    * Patients with mantle zone pattern may have better survival.[2]
* Bone marrow involvement can have different patterns; making a diagnosis of MCL solely based on BM is not recommended.

Immunophenotype

* B-cell antigens (CD19, CD20, CD22), surface IgM with or without IgD strongly positive, lambda light chain predominates, bcl-2 positive

- CD5 positive, CD10 negative, CD23 negative, FMC7 positive
- Nuclear cyclin D1 stain is positive—pathognomonic.
  - Note that cyclin D1 staining is difficult to perform and may be unreliable; fluorescence in situ hybridization (FISH) testing may be helpful to ascertain the diagnosis.
- Blastoid variants have higher proliferative index (Ki-67 or MIB-1).
- Prominent meshworks of follicular dendritic cells (CD21 positive, CD35 positive)
- MCL with GI involvement expresses gut-specific adhesion receptor $\alpha 4/\beta 7$ integrin.

Cytogenetic and Molecular Changes

- Ig genes rearranged; IgV genes unmutated (pregerminal center origin) in about 80% of cases, with increased frequency of specific IgVH genes
- t(11;14) in 70% on conventional cytogenetics and almost 100% on FISH
- The translocation is between CYCLIN D1 (also known as CCND1, BCL-1, or PRAD1) and IgH.
  - Cyclin D1 protein is involved in cell cycle control at G1 phase and is not normally expressed in lymphocytes.
  - Cyclin D1 can come in "a" and "b" isoforms; cyclin D1a has both cytoplasmic and nuclear localization and is thought to be less oncogenic than cyclin D1b isoform which is only nuclear; in vivo, short cyclin D1a isoforms may play a greater role than cycline D1b isoforms.
  - Both existence of cyclin D1-negative MCL and of t(11;14) in other lymphomas is controversial.
    - Recent analysis of six cases of truly cyclin D1-negative MCL-lacking t(11;14) by FISH found them to have cyclin D2 and D3 expression.[3]
      - This appears to be a very rare exception to the rule requiring cyclin D1 positivity for the diagnosis.
    - There is t(11;14) in a subset of multiple myeloma but with a different IgH breakpoint.
- CYCLIN D1 gene is necessary but not sufficient to develop MCL, because additional mutations are present more than 90% of the time.

- Inactivating mutations in cell cycle controllers such as cyclin-dependent kinase inhibitors p16 and p17 and decrease in p27 expression (greater than 50%)
  - Inactivation of ATM gene, which is located on 11q22 and is involved in DNA double-strand break repair, in 40–50%
- Blastoid variant is associated with greater number of cytogenetic abnormalities, higher proportion of p16 and p53 inactivation, and increased incidence of tetraploidy with higher incidence of centrosome abnormalities (this is particularly true of pleomorphic blastoid variant).
- Leukemic phase MCL is associated with 8q negative.
- Several gene-expression profiles revealed not only involvement of cell cycle control genes, but also up-regulation of multidrug resistance, NFκB pathway, and anti-apoptosis genes.[4,5]
- Overall, adverse prognosis is conferred by high proliferation index (Ki-67 or MIB-1); inactivation of DNA damage repair by mutation of p53 and p14 and over-expression of MDM2; loss of negative cell cycle regulators p16, p18, p21 and p27; over-expression of positive cell cycle regulator cdk4, BMI-1, and cdk1; and anti-apoptotic over-expression of bcl-2 and loss of Bim.

■ Prognosis

- IPI on the whole is not prognostic, whereas poor PS and age older than 60 years are.
- Follicular Lymphoma International Prognostic Index appears more predictive than IPI.[6]
- Other clinical adverse factors include advanced stage, splenomegaly, anemia, and lymphocytosis.
- Pathologic adverse factors include peripheral blood involvement, β2-microglobulin greater than 3mg/L, blastoid variant, high proliferation index, low p27 levels, p53 mutations, and greater than five chromosomal aberrations.
- Mantle zone pattern and VH3-21/VL3-19 phenotype are prognostically better.

■ Treatment

Treatment of Early Stage (I/II) Disease

* Unusual, only 10–15% of cases
* Retrospective review of 26 patients with stages IA and IIA had 17 patients treated with involved field radiation therapy with or without chemotherapy and 9 with chemotherapy or observation.[7]
  * Five-year progression-free survival (PFS) was 46%; OS was 70%, with five patients surviving more than 8 years.
  * Patients younger than 60 and those receiving radiation therapy had better outcomes.

Treatment of Advanced Stage (III/IV) Disease

* No standard therapy prolongs survival.
* Multiagent chemotherapy in general yields overall response rate (ORR) of 40–90%, complete remission (CR) 20–30%, with response duration of 8–12 months.
* Regimens incorporating anthracyclines have higher CR by 10–20%, but do not affect any outcome measures.
* Single-agent fludarabine: ORR 30–70%, CR about 30% (similar to cyclophosphamide, doxorubicin, and prednisone [CHOP])
* Single-agent rituximab: ORR 27%, CR 2%, with no benefit to prolonged infusion.[8]
* Chemoimmunotherapy:
  * CHOP vs. R-CHOP: Lenz et al. randomized 122 untreated patients to six cycles of R-CHOP or CHOP followed by second randomization to autologous stem cell transplantation (ASCT) if younger than 65 years old or interferon (IFN) maintenance (Figure 5-1).
    * ORR improved from 75% to 94%, CR from 7% to 34%, TTF from 14 to 21 months without a difference in PFS or OS (77% at 2 years).[9]
  * FCM vs. R-FCM: in 48 relapsed patients first randomized to four cycles of therapy and then randomized to two courses of rituximab or observation, initial addition of rituximab improved ORR from 46% to 58% and CR from 0% to 29%, without statistically significant changes in PFS (4 vs. 8 months) (Figure 5-2).

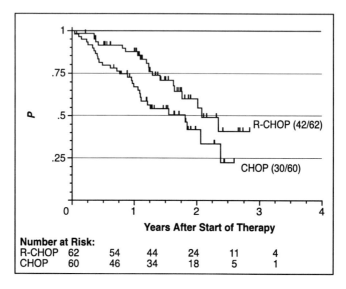

Figure 5-1: Median time to initiation of salvage therapy following cyclophosphamide, doxorubicin, vincristine, and prednisone (CHOP) and rituximab and CHOP (R-CHOP). Patients assigned to R-CHOP experienced a significantly longer time to salvage therapy (P=.0262). G. Lenz et al: *J Clin Oncol;* 2005:1984–1992. Used with permission from ASCO.

- There was a statistically significant improvement in median OS from 11 months to not reached (P=.004), with estimated OS going from 35% to 65% at 2 years. These data have not matured enough to determine if the regimen changed the natural history of the disease.[10]
- Subsequent randomization to rituximab maintenance (four weekly doses at 3 and 9 months) showed that it did not improve median remission duration (14 vs. 12 months) but improved proportion of remissions beyond 2 years (45% vs. 9%).[11]
- Aggressive chemotherapy: hyper-CVAD/M-A
  - An intensive regimen pioneered at MD Anderson for highly aggressive lymphomas/ALL that may result in survival prolongation
  - Consists of eight treatments with two combinations alternating every 3 weeks: hyperfractionated cy-

B

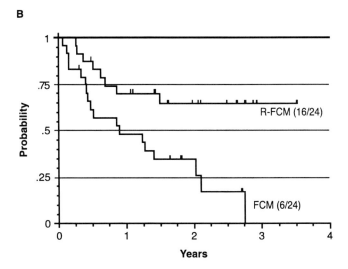

Figure 5-2: Overall survival after start of therapy for patients with mantle cell lymphoma (MCL) randomized for FCM or R-FCM. Used with permission from *Blood,* Journal of the American Society of Hematology. Forstpointner, R., 2004, Vol. 104, Issue 10, 3064–3071. Figure 3B.

clophosphamide with mesna, vincristine, doxorubicin, and dexamethasone and methotrexate with cytarabine
* Original study showed that when used prior to ASCT in 43 untreated and relapsed patients, hyper-CVAD/M-A had ORR of 94% and CR of 38%.
  * Untreated patients had significantly better 3-year event-free survival (EFS) of 72% and OS of 92%.
* In an update of 33 untreated patients, demonstrated 5-year DFS of 43% and OS of 77%.[12]
* Addition of rituximab to hyper-CVAD/M-A used without subsequent ASCT in 97 untreated patients yielded CR/CRu of 87%, 3-year FFS of 67% and OS of 81%.[13]
  * The regimen was toxic, with TRM and MDS/AML resulting in 8% mortality.
* Kahl et al. modified R-hyper-CVAD by omitting M-A and administered it to 22 patients with newly diagnosed MCL, followed by rituximab maintenance (4 doses every 6 months for 2 years) in responders.

- Two patients died before restaging, prompting protocol modification and no further deaths.
- Seventy-seven percent of the remaining patients achieved CR/CRu.
- With median follow-up of 37 months, 2-year PFS was 59% and OS was 77%, only slightly inferior to unmodified R-hyperCVAD/M-A.[14]
- Authors speculate that median PFS of 37 months was due to inclusion of maintenance rituximab; however, the role of maintenance rituximab in MCL is far from clear (see maintenance rituximab after R-FCM as mentioned above).
- Dose-adjusted EPOCH (etoposide, prednisone, vincristine, cyclophosphamide, doxorubicin) combined with rituximab in 26 patients achieved 92% CR and, following idiotype vaccination, resulted in OS of 89% at median follow-up of 46 months, with median EFS of 22 months.[15]
- Autologous transplantation
  - Because MCL is chemosensitive but quickly relapses, ASCT was attempted to improve duration remission and possibly survival.
  - The largest retrospective review included 195 patients, with overall 2-year OS of 76% and 5-year OS of 50%.
    - Median survival of 59 months compared favorably with typical survival duration.
    - Patients transplanted in first CR, however, had 2-year OS of 88% and 5-year OS of 65%, with transplantation beyond first CR having a hazard ratio of 2.95.[16]
  - Prospective European MCL network trial randomized 122 newly diagnosed patients who responded to CHOP-like induction regimen (25% with rituximab) to ASCT vs. IFN maintenance (Figure 5-3).
    - CHOP-like induction did not achieve a remission in 23% of the initial group of 230. Of evaluable responders, 32% had CR (17% by intention to treat).
    - As compared to IFN group, ASCT group had improved 3-year PFS from 25% to 54%, without significant improvement in 3-year OS (77 vs. 83%).[17]

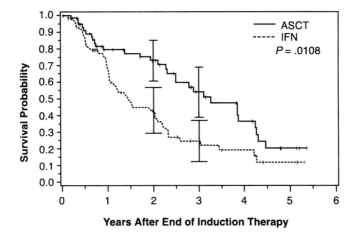

Number at Risk:

ASCT	62	38	31	17	10	3
IFN	60	33	19	9	6	2

Figure 5-3: Progression-free survival after high-dose radiochemother-apy followed by autologous stem cell transplantation (ASCT) and inter-feron-α (IFN) maintenance in MCL. Patients assigned to stem cell transplantation experience significantly longer progression-free survival (log-rank test). Vertical bars indicate 95% confidence intervals for progression-free survival. Used with permission from *Blood,* Journal of the American Society of Hematology. Dreyling, M, Vol. 105, Issue 7, 2677–2684, April 1, 2006.

- ASCT thus appears more beneficial in first CR, but optimal induction regimen, high-dose chemotherapy (HDC), and need for in vivo purging of stem cells with rituximab remain unclear.
  - One series noted improved 4-year DFS (68% vs. 33%, p=0.02) with hyper-CVAD as compared to CHOP-like induction regimen.[18]
  - DHAP, also an intensive regimen, has been used successfully to salvage CHOP induction failures pre-ASCT, with 84% CR, 3-year EFS of 83% and OS of 90%.[19]
  - Four to six cycles of R-DHAP followed by ASCT in patients under 60 years of age resulted in a similar 3 year EFS of 76% and OS of 75%.[20]

■ At Memorial Sloan-Kettering Cancer Center (MSKCC), 46 patients with untreated MCL received CHOP-14 or similar regimen followed by ICE, with or without rituximab, followed by ASCT, resulting in 80% CR, estimated 5-year PFS of 58%, and 5-year OS of 83%.[21]

■ While rituximab given at any point can be considered "in vivo purging," it most commonly refers to rituximab given during HDC before stem cell collection.

  • Twenty-eight untreated patients who received CHOP-like treatment followed by sequential HDC incorporating rituximab achieved CR in 100% with one toxic death, 4.5-year EFS of 79%, and OS of 89%.[22]

  • Twenty untreated patients treated with CHOP had rituximab before stem collection and after ASCT, with 3 year PFS of 89% and OS 88%.[23]

    ■ Small studies demonstrate increased molecular remission rate after post-ASCT rituximab.

  • Both studies showed improvement in survival over historical controls receiving conventional chemotherapy without ASCT.

■ Allogeneic transplantation

  • Full-dose allo-SCT has decreased relapse but increased treatment-related mortality (TRM), resulting in the same OS as ASCT.

  • Nonmyeloablative ("mini") allo-ASCT may reduce TRM and is promising as per two single-institution trials.

    ■ Thirty-three relapsed patients, 42% after ASCT, had related (49%) or unrelated mini-allo-stem cell transplantation (SCT) with CR of 75%, 2-year DFS of 60%, and OS of 65%, still with a significant 2-year TRM of 24%.[24]

    ■ In 18 patients who were prognostically better (89% chemosensitive disease, only 28% relapsed after ASCT), mini-allo-SCT resulted in CR of 94%, 3-year EFS of 82%, and OS of 86%, with minimal TRM of 6%.[25]

- Registry data on mini-allo-ASCT included 22 patients with MCL who had horrific outcomes with extreme toxicity, resulting in 2-year TRM of 82%, PFS of 0%, and OS of 13%.[26]
- Radioimmunotherapy
  - Targeted radiation therapy via radiolabeled anti-CD20 antibodies provides additional means of treatment with reduced systemic toxicity.
  - It can be used in patients not eligible for ASCT or as part of conditioning pre-ASCT.
    - MSKCC has recently completed a trial of 131I-labeled anti-CD20 antibody tositumomab (Bexxar) followed by CHOP in 24 patients with untreated MCL who were not eligible for ASCT, with preliminary results showing 75% CR rate.
    - A trial of 16 patients with relapsed MCL treated with higher dose of Bexxar followed by HDC/ASCT has shown 73% CR, 3-year PFS of 61%, and 3-year OS of 93%, without any treatment-related deaths.[27]
- Proteasome inhibitors: bortezomib
  - Bortezomib is a boronic-acid inhibitor of 26S proteasome; this inhibition is thought to prevent degradation of cell cycle inhibitors such as p27 and of NFκB pathway inhibitor IκB.
  - In two simultaneously published small phase II trials, there was a significant response.
  - A follow-up multicenter phase II trial of 155 patients showed ORR of 38% and CR/CRu of 8%, with median duration of response of 9 months and time to progression of 6 months.
  - One-year OS was 69% with median follow-up of 13 months.[28]

General Treatment Approach

- Clinical trial at any point and stage of treatment
- Early stage disease
  - CHOP-like chemotherapy, with or without rituximab, and IFRT.

- Advanced stage disease
  - If transplant eligible:
    - Four cycles of R-CHOP, two cycles of R-ICE or R-DHAP, and ASCT, or
    - Six cycles of R-hyper-CVAD/M-A or of modified R-hyper-CVAD, and ASCT
    - Six cycles of R-hyper-CVAD/M-A without ASCT may also be considered.
  - If not transplant eligible:
    - If good PS, six cycles of R-hyper-CVAD/M-A
    - If poor PS, R-CVP, R-CHOP, or modified R-hyper-CVAD
- Relapsed disease
  - If transplant eligible: ASCT or mini-allo-SCT.
  - If not transplant eligible, R-FCM could be considered.
  - Consider radioimmunotherapy or bortezomib in either case.

■ References

1. Fisher RI, Dahlberg S, Nathwani BN, et al. A clinical analysis of two indolent lymphoma entities: mantle cell lymphoma and marginal zone lymphoma (including the mucosa-associated lymphoid tissue and monocytoid B-cell subcategories): a Southwest Oncology Group study. *Blood.* 1995;85:1075–1082.

2. Majlis A, Pugh WC, Rodriguez MA, et al. Mantle cell lymphoma: correlation of clinical outcome and biologic features with three histologic variants. *J Clin Oncol.* 1997;15(4): 1664–1671.

3. Fu K, Weisenburger DD, Greiner TC, et al. Cyclin D1-negative mantle cell lymphoma: a clinicopathologic study based on gene expression profiling. *Blood.* 2005;106:4315–4321.

4. Rosenwald A, Wright G, Wiestner A, et al. The proliferation gene expression signature is a quantitative integrator of oncogenic events that predicts survival in mantle cell lymphoma. *Cancer Cell.* 2003;3:185–197.

5. Thieblemont C, Nasser V, Felman P, et al. Small lymphocytic lymphoma, marginal zone B-cell lymphoma, and mantle cell lymphoma exhibit distinct gene-expression profiles allowing molecular diagnosis. *Blood.* 2004;103:2727–2737.

6. Moller MB, Pedersen NT, Christensen BE. Mantle cell lymphoma: prognostic capacity of the Follicular Lymphoma International Prognostic Index. *Br J Haematol.* 2006; 133(1):43–49.

7. Leitch HA, Gascoyne RD, Chhanabhai M, et al. Limited-stage mantle-cell lymphoma. *Ann Oncol.* 2003;14:1555–1561.

8. Ghielmini M, Schmitz SF, Cogliatti S, et al. Effect of single-agent rituximab given at the standard schedule or as prolonged treatment in patients with mantle cell lymphoma: a study of the Swiss Group for Clinical Cancer Research (SAKK). *J Clin Oncol.* 2005;23(4):705–711.

9. Lenz G, Dreyling M, Hoster E, et al. Immunochemotherapy with rituximab and cyclophosphamide, doxorubicin, vincristine, and prednisone significantly improves response and time to treatment failure, but not long-term outcome in patients with previously untreated mantle cell lymphoma: results of a prospective randomized trial of the German Low Grade Lymphoma Study Group (GLSG). *J Clin Oncol.* 2005;23:1984–1992.

10. Forstpointner R, Dreyling M, Repp R, et al. The addition of rituximab to a combination of fludarabine, cyclophosphamide, mitoxantrone (FCM) significantly increases the response rate and prolongs survival as compared with FCM alone in patients with relapsed and refractory follicular and mantle cell lymphomas: results of a prospective randomized study of the German Low-Grade Lymphoma Study Group. *Blood.* 2004;104:3064–3071.

11. Forstpointner R, Unterhalt M, Dreyling M, et al. Maintenance therapy with rituximab leads to a significant prolongation of response duration after salvage therapy with a combination of rituximab, fludarabine, cyclophosphamide, and mitoxantrone (R-FCM) in patients with recurring and refractory follicular and mantle cell lymphomas: Results of a prospective randomized study of the German Low Grade Lymphoma Study Group (GLSG). *Blood.* 2006;108(13): 4003–4008.

12. Khouri IF, Saliba RM, Okoroji GJ, et al. Long-term follow-up of autologous stem cell transplantation in patients with diffuse mantle cell lymphoma in first disease remission: the prognostic value of beta2-microglobulin and the tumor score. *Cancer.* 2003;98:2630–2635.

13. Romaguera JE, Fayad L, Rodriguez MA, et al. High rate of durable remissions after treatment of newly diagnosed

aggressive mantle-cell lymphoma with rituximab plus hyper-CVAD alternating with rituximab plus high-dose methotrexate and cytarabine. *J Clin Oncol.* 2005;23(28):7013–7023.

14. Kahl B, Longo W, Eickhoff J, et al. Maintenance rituximab following induction chemoimmunotherapy may prolong progression-free survival in mantle cell lymphoma: a pilot study from the Wisconsin Oncology Network. *Ann Oncol.* 2006; 17:1418–1423.

15. Neelapu SS, Kwak LW, Kobrin CB, et al. Vaccine-induced tumor-specific immunity despite severe B-cell depletion in mantle cell lymphoma. *Nat Med.* 2005;11:986–991.

16. Vandenberghe E, Ruiz de Elvira C, Loberiza FR, et al. Outcome of autologous transplantation for mantle cell lymphoma: a study by the European Blood and Bone Marrow Transplant and Autologous Blood and Marrow Transplant Registries. *Br J Haematol.* 2003;120:793–800.

17. Dreyling M, Lenz G, Hoster E, et al. Early consolidation by myeloablative radiochemotherapy followed by autologous stem cell transplantation in first remission significantly prolongs progression-free survival in mantle-cell lymphoma: results of a prospective randomized trial of the European MCL Network. *Blood.* 2005;105:2677–2684.

18. Conde E, Marco F, Caballero D, et al. Autologous Stem Cell Transplantation (ASCT) for Mantle Cell Lymphoma (MCL). *Blood.* 2002;100:2529a.

19. Lefrere F, Delmer A, Suzan F, et al. Sequential chemotherapy by CHOP and DHAP regimens followed by high-dose therapy with stem cell transplantation induces a high rate of complete response and improves event-free survival in mantle cell lymphoma: a prospective study. *Leukemia.* 2002; 16(4):587–593.

20. de Guibert S, Jaccard A, Bernard M, Turlure P, Bordessoule D, Lamy T. Rituximab and DHAP followed by intensive therapy with autologous stem-cell transplantation as first-line therapy for mantle cell lymphoma. *Haematologica.* 2006;91(3):425–426.

21. Persky D, Portlock CS, Lessac-Chenen S, et al. The Utility of Consolidative Upfront High Dose Chemoradiotherapy and ASCT in Patients with Mantle Cell Lymphoma (MCL). *Blood.* 2005;106(11):2072a.

22. Gianni AM, Magni M, Martelli M, et al: Long-term remission in mantle cell lymphoma following high-dose sequential chemotherapy and in vivo rituximab-purged stem cell autografting (R-HDS regimen). *Blood.* 2003;102:749–755.

23. Mangel J, Leitch HA, Connors JM, et al. Intensive chemotherapy and autologous stem-cell transplantation plus rituximab is superior to conventional chemotherapy for newly diagnosed advanced stage mantle-cell lymphoma: a matched pair analysis. *Ann Oncol.* 2004;15(2):283–290.

24. Maris MB, Sandmaier BM, Storer BE, et al: Allogeneic hematopoietic cell transplantation after fludarabine and 2 Gy total body irradiation for relapsed and refractory mantle cell lymphoma. *Blood.* 2004;104:3535–3542.

25. Khouri IF, Saliba RM, Okoroji GJ, et al. Long-term follow-up of autologous stem cell transplantation in patients with diffuse mantle cell lymphoma in first disease remission: the prognostic value of beta2-microglobulin and the tumor score. *Cancer.* 2003;98(12):2630–2635.

26. Robinson SP, Goldstone AH, Mackinnon S, et al. Chemoresistant or aggressive lymphoma predicts for a poor outcome following reduced-intensity allogeneic progenitor cell transplantation: an analysis from the Lymphoma Working Party of the European Group for Blood and Bone Marrow Transplantation. *Blood.* 2002;100(13):4310–4316.

27. Gopal AK, Rajendran JG, Petersdorf SH, et al: High-dose chemo-radioimmunotherapy with autologous stem cell support for relapsed mantle cell lymphoma. *Blood.* 2002;99: 3158–3162.

28. Fisher RI, Bernstein SH, Kahl BS, et al. Multicenter phase II study of bortezomib in patients with relapsed or refractory mantle cell lymphoma. *J Clin Oncol.* 2006;24(30):4867–4874.

CHAPTER 6

Hodgkin's Lymphoma

■ Epidemiology

* The term Hodgkin's disease initially was used because of the uncertainty of whether this entity was a tumor or an infection. By the late 1990s, evidence showed that the Hodgkin Reed-Sternberg cell is a B cell; thus the term Hodgkin's lymphoma (HL) is more appropriate.

* It has one of the best survivals of all lymphomas—over 80% at 5 years. Most research is aimed at stratifying treatment to match disease severity, particularly to minimize long-term toxicity in low-risk patients.

* Approximately 8,190 new cases of HL are estimated for 2007, about one-eighth of NHL, with 1,070 estimated deaths.

* Incidence rates have been stable over the last 20 years.

* Slight male predominance (1.4 to 1) and bimodal distribution for age of onset, with the first larger peak in the 20s and the second in the 50s to 60s.
  * Second peak is smaller in modern series, likely as a result of better diagnostic capabilities.

* Nodular sclerosis (NS) is the most common histologic subtype.

* Increased incidence in first-degree relatives (two- to fivefold), particularly siblings of younger, but not older, adults with HL (sevenfold), same-sex siblings (ninefold) and identical twins (100-fold).

* Association with particular human leukocyte antigen (HLA) haplotypes, especially HLA-A1, and low-secreting genotype for IL-6 (high IL-6 levels are prognostically poor in HL).

* Association with Epstein-Barr Virus (EBV):
  * Higher incidence of HL is correlated with low socioeconomic status and with living in a developing country;

the first peak is in childhood, suggesting an infectious etiology, with mixed cellularity (MC) being the most common histologic subtype.

- Several-fold increase in the risk of HL after acute EBV infection (infectious mononucleosis [IM]).
- EBV-positive and negative cases of HL have different age distributions, with EBV-negative cases having a unimodal age distribution in young adulthood.
- Hjalgrim et al. compared incidence rates of HL in three population-based cohorts (two Danish and one Swedish) of patients who were tested for IM, for a total of 38,555 patients with serologic evidence of IM.
  - Only serologically confirmed IM was associated with an increased incidence of HL.
  - Sixteen of 29 tumors obtained from patients with a history of IM had evidence of EBV. There was no evidence of an increased risk of EBV-negative HL after IM.
  - The relative risk for EBV-positive HL after IM was 4.0, and the median incubation time from IM to HL was only 4.1 years.[1]
- Patients presenting with HL subsequent to EBV infection may have had a more severe infection, with elevated titers against viral capsid antigen and EBV nuclear antigens compared to controls.
- Latent membrane protein 1, an EBV-latent gene that is highly expressed in Hodgkin and Reed-Sternberg (HRS) cells, can induce B cell activation markers as well as IL-10 production, up-regulate several anti-apoptosis genes, including bcl-2, and appears to function as a constitutively activated tumor necrosis factor receptor and as a result can activate a variety of signaling pathways, including NFκB.
- Association with immune suppression:
  - HL risk increases 7.6-fold in patients with human immunodeficiency virus (HIV), where it is almost always EBV-positive and can occur with relatively preserved CD4 counts.
  - Increased risk after transplantation, occurring more than 4 years out.

■ Presentation

- HL typically spreads from cervical lymph nodes sequentially down the lymph node chains over a period of months.
  - Due to this pattern, it would be unusual to see disease in lower lymph node chains, such as in the abdomen, without disease in the neck.
  - Liver and bone marrow are typically involved after spleen; lungs after ipsilateral hilar lymph nodes.
  - This is particularly true for NS and MC, and less so for lymphocyte-depleted (LD) and lymphocyte-rich (LR) histologic subtypes.
- Presents as painless lymphadenopathy in about 70%
  - Sixty to 80% of those in cervical or supraclavicular areas, mediastinum 50–60%, paraaortic area 30–40%, axilla 20–40%, less in lower lymph node chains.
  - Lymph nodes typically feel small, mobile, and rubbery ("beebees").
- Other presentations include incidental mediastinal mass and nonspecific systemic symptoms.
- B symptoms in about 25%, more common in advanced stage disease
- Diffuse pruritus in 10–15%, may precede the diagnosis by months
- In rare cases, there is pain after ingestion of alcohol, usually at the sites of involvement.
- Extranodal disease 10–15%, most commonly lung and bone, less commonly liver and bone marrow (5–7%), and rare central nervous system and gastrointestinal (GI) involvement.
- Paraneoplastic syndromes are extremely rare and include neurologic syndromes, nephrotic syndrome, and hypercalcemia.
- Blood tests may show normocytic anemia and eosinophilia.
- Staging workup:
  - Excisional lymph node biopsy is preferred for adequate tissue. Inguinal lymph nodes and extranodal sites are lower yield. Suspicious extranodal sites should be biopsied for staging.

- Cotswolds meeting in 1988 made recommendations for the workup to include:
  - History and physical (with focus on B symptoms); chest X-ray; computerized tomography (CT) of chest, abdomen, and pelvis; complete blood count with lymphocyte count; erythrocyte sedimentation rate (ESR); liver function tests; albumin; lactate dehydrogenase; calcium; and bone marrow biopsy except for stages IA/IIA.
- Patients with stage IA/IIA disease without anemia/leucopenia; stage IA/IIA younger than 35 years old, with either anemia or leucopenia but without inguinal/iliac involvement, or stage IIIA/IV without any risk factors may be spared bone marrow (BM) biopsy based on a clinical prediction rule where their risk of BM involvement was estimated at 0.3%.[2]
- HIV testing if risk factors or unusual presentation are seen.
- Gallium scan could help in differentiating between mediastinal residual disease and fibrosis after treatment. It is being replaced by positron emission tomography (PET), which is more sensitive and provides better resolution, particularly in the abdomen.
  - PET is often obtained at baseline for staging, and after completion of therapy to confirm complete remission.
- Bone scans, ultrasound, and magnetic resonance imaging in selected cases.
- Staging laparotomy and lymphangiography are not recommended due to modern imaging techniques and treatment modalities. Laparatomy could still have utility in early stage HL if treatment with radiation therapy (RT) only is considered.
- Staging: Due to sequential disease spread, Cotswolds modification of Ann Arbor staging system is excellent for HL, for which it was originally designed.
- Restaging after initial treatment:
  - Most patients with HL will have a residual mass on CT scan following the completion of initial therapy.

- A mass may contain fibrosis, necrotic tissue, residual HL, or an unsuspected concurrent diffuse large B-cell lymphoma (DLBCL).
- CT scans cannot differentiate post-treatment fibrosis from active disease.
- CT scans have limited utility in discerning active disease in normal size lymph nodes or in some extranodal sites, particularly bone.
- Functional imaging with PET scans improves sensitivity in detecting of active HL.
- The major problem with PET scanning is the high rate of false positives.
- PET scan has both high positive predictive value (PPV; positive PET result in a patient who has a subsequent relapse) and high negative predictive value (NPV; negative PET result in a patient who is progression free).
  - In a recent prospective trial, PET scan after two cycles of treatment was predictive of both progression-free survival (PFS) and overall survival (OS), with calculated PPV of 69% and NPV of 95%.[3]
- PET scan has considerable utility in post-treatment, more than pretreatment, evaluation.
- Due to high false-positive rate of PET scanning, if the PET scan is positive after therapy, the most PET-avid accessible lesion should be biopsied.
- If a PET scan is normal, monitoring of any size residual mass by CT scans is warranted.

■ Pathology

Morphology

- Neoplastic HRS cells comprise less than 2% of the lymph node, admixed with a major population of B cells, T cells, plasma cells, eosinophils, neutrophils, histiocytes, and stromal cells.
- Two major types exist, with immunophenotype being very helpful for differentiation:
  - Ninety-five percent have classical HL (cHL), with four histologic subtypes: NS, MC, LR, and LD.

- Neoplastic HRS cells are large, with abundant cytoplasm, have bilobed or multiple large nuclei, and prominent eosinophilic nucleolus in each of at least two nuclear lobes.
- They express the activation markers CD30 and CD15 and usually lack CD45 and B lineage antigens.
  - Five percent have nodular lymphocyte predominant HL (NLPHL).
    - Tumor cells are L&H (lymphocytic and histiocytic) HRS cell variants, also called "popcorn cells" due to bulging nuclei that resemble popped corn.
    - B cell markers are expressed and CD30 and CD15 are absent.
    - It is clinically a different disease with its own disease course. Prognosis and treatment and will be discussed separately.
- Nodular sclerosis (NS) (60–80%): as the name implies, a nodular pattern is separated by sclerotic fibrous tissue. HRS cells are "lacunar," owing to receding cytoplasm due to preparation artifact.
  - Some investigators grade NS as 1 or 2, with grade 2 showing clusters or sheets of lacunar cells in at least 25% of the nodules. It is questionable whether the outcome of NS grade 2 is worse, particularly with modern treatment.
- Mixed cellularity (15–30%): Significant sclerosis is absent, but vague nodular pattern and thin fibrotic bands may still be present.
  - As compared to NS, MC less frequently involves mediastinum and affects at least as many women as men.
- Lymphocyte-rich (5%): lymphocytic infiltrate and paucity of eosinophils characterizes this subgroup.
  - It can be nodular but is distinguished from NLPHL by cHL immunophenotype. Prognostically it also is closer to cHL than NHPHL.
- Lymphocyte depleted (less than 1%): diffuse pattern with many HRS cells, extensive fibrosis, and few reactive cells. Its reticular variant, with sheets of HRS cells, is difficult to distinguish from anaplastic large cell lymphoma.

* More prevalent in HIV-positive patients, presents at older age and more advanced stage[4]

Immunophenotype

* CD30 positive in virtually all cases; CD15 positive in 85%
* No B-cell antigens except for CD20 in up to one-third, which may be prognostically worse; no T-cell antigens

Cytogenetic and Molecular Changes

* In the last 10 years, HL has been proven to be a clonal B-cell germinal-center-derived lymphoma through a combination of micromanipulation of HRS cells from frozen samples and polymerase chain reaction amplification of genes from these single cells.[5, 6]
* Immunoglobulin (Ig) genes are rearranged, consistent with germinal- or post-germinal-center B cell origin, but are not expressed, with evidence that promoters and enhancers of Ig genes are not activated and downstream signaling is decreased, without detectable mRNA.
  * Notable absence of other markers of germinal-center origin, such as bcl-6 or CD10.
* Somatic mutations are also present but render original Ig variable region rearrangements nonfunctional (crippling mutations); despite this, HRS cells somehow avoid apoptosis, possibly due to constitutive NFκB activation. After transformation, there is no evidence of ongoing somatic hypermutation.
* Occasional patients with both HL and NHL frequently show identical Ig gene rearrangements and somatic mutations in HRS and NHL cells, suggesting same clonal origin.
* Aneuploidy and frequent 14q abnormalities but without typical aberrations.

■ Prognosis

* For early stage (I/II) disease (ESHL), poor prognostic factors, as based on all the criteria used by three trial groups, are age older than 50, B symptoms or ESR

greater than 50, bulky disease defined as any mass over 10 cm or large mediastinal adenopathy (LMA), extranodal disease, and at least three to four sites of lymph node involvement above the diaphragm.

- Cotswolds' definition of LMA is more than one-third (or 0.35) of internal thoracic diameter at T5/6 interspace, whereas Ann Arbor's is more than one-third of greatest intrathoracic diameter. Either definition may be used.
- Other established risk factors not included in the criteria are male gender, mixed-cellularity or lymphocyte-depleted histology, and infradiaphragmatic disease.
- Earlier studies used age cutoff of 40 years.
- Possible risk factors also include eosinophilia in nodular sclerosis Hodgkin's lymphoma.
- Using prognostic criteria, three groups of early stage patients are usually defined: very favorable, favorable, and unfavorable ESHL (Table 6-1).
- Very favorable ESHL (stage IA, upper-cervical lymph nodes, no risk factors) accounts for only 5% of cases and is usually treated with minimal RT alone.
  - With no specific randomized studies addressing this cohort of patients, it will not be discussed further.
- Historically, patients with stage I or II HL with favorable prognostic features were candidates for primary RT or short combined modality therapy (CMT), whereas patients with unfavorable prognostic factors tended to receive full-course CMT.
- German Hodgkin's Lymphoma Study Group (GHSG) treats stage IIB w/ LMA or extranodal disease as advanced stage.
- For advanced stage (III/IV) disease (ASHL), poor prognostic factors as based on a study of 5,141 patients are age 45 or older, male, stage IV vs. III disease, serum albumin less than 4g/dl, hemoglobin less than 10.5 mg/dl, white blood cell count greater than or equal to 15,000/mm3, and absolute lymphocyte count less than 600/mm3 (or less than 8% of total white blood cell count).

**Table 6-1: Risk Factors and Treatment Groups in Early
Stage Hodgkin's Lymphoma (ESHL)**

*EORTC Risk factors	*GHSG	**NCCN
A. Large MM	A. Large MM	A. Large MM/any >10 cm
B. Age ≥50 years	B. Extranodal disease	
C. ESR ≥50 (or ≥30 with B symptoms	C. ESR ≥50 (or ≥30 with B symptoms	C. B symptoms (or ESR ≥50 if asymptomatic)
D. ≥4 involved sites	D. ≥3 involved sites	D. ≥ 4 involved sites
Treatment groups		
Early Stage Favorable	CS I-II with no RF	CS I-II with no RF
Early Stage Unfavorable	CS I-II with any RF	CS I, CSIIA with any RF; CSIIB with C/D but without A/B
Advanced Stage	CS III-IV	CS IIB with A/B; CS III-IV

Abbreviations: CS = clinical stage; EORTC = European Organization for
Research and Treatment of Cancer; GHSG = German Hodgkin's
Lymphoma Study Group; MM = mediastinal mass; NCCN = National
Comprehensive Cancer Network; RF = risk factors.
*Adapted from Diehl V, Thomas RK, Re D. Part II: Hodgkin's lymphoma—
diagnosis and treatment. *Lancet Oncol* 2004;5(1):19-26.
**Data from: NCCN Clinical Practice Guidelines in Oncology: Hodgkin
Disease/Lymphoma V. I. 2006. Available at www.nccn.org/professionals/
physicians_gls/PDF/hodgkins. pdf. Accessed April 6, 2007.

- These seven factors (mnemonic *WALSHAM*) make
  up the international prognostic score (IPS) developed
  by Hasenclever et al.[7] (Table 6-2).
- Based on IPS, patients can be divided into three risk
  groups (Figure 6-1):
  - IPS score of 0-2 (low risk) represents 58% of
    ASHL, with 5-year freedom from progression
    (FFP) rate of 74% and OS of 86%.

**Table 6-2:   International Prognostic Score (IPS) for
                Advanced Stage Hodgkin's Lymphoma (ASHL)**

WBC $\geq 15,000/mm^3$
Albumin (serum) <4 g/dl
Lymphocyte count $<600/mm^3$ (or $<8\%$ of WBC)
Stage IV
Hemoglobin <10.5 g/dl
Age ≥ 45
Male

Number of risk factors	Percent patients in each group	5-yr FFP (%)	5-yr OS (%)
0–1	29	84	89
2	29	67	81
3	23	60	78
4–7	19	47	59

Abbreviation: FFP = freedom from progression
Data from: Hasenclever et al, *NEJM* 1998.

- IPS score of 3 (intermediate risk) accounts for 23% of ASHL, with FFP of 60% and OS of 78%.
- IPS score of 4 or more (high risk) accounting for only 19% of ASHL, with FFP of 47% and OS of 59%.
- Chemotherapy for patients with high-risk IPS may be intensified, as done by GSHG.

■ Treatment

Treatment of Early Stage Disease (ESHL)

- Standard approach is controversial, because patients who relapse have excellent outcome regardless of the initial treatment strategy, resulting in the same OS rates.
  - RT alone—to avoid chemotherapy, which can be reserved for patients who fail RT

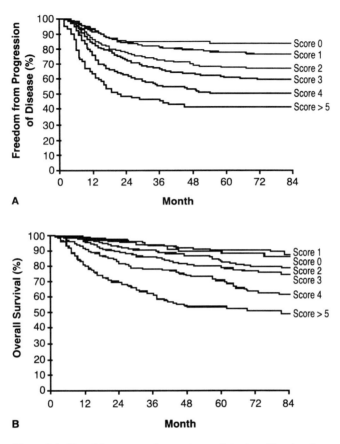

Figure 6-1: Use of the prognostic score to predict rates of freedom from progression of disease (Panel A) and overall survival (Panel B) in 1,618 patients with advanced Hodgkin's disease. Hasenclever et al. *NEJM* 339(21): 1506–1514, Figure 1, Nov. 1998. Used with permission.

- CMT: The number of chemotherapy cycles as well as the RT fields continues to be reduced. Proponents argue that disease control is best with this approach despite the fact that patients who fail need to receive autologous stem cell transplantation (ASCT).
- The aims of multicenter randomized clinical trials in ESHL are to decrease the number of chemotherapy cycles, avoid leukemogenic chemotherapeutic agents,

reduce the dose of RT, decrease the size of the RT field, or eliminate RT altogether.

- A recent trend is to use full-course chemotherapy alone to decrease the incidence of secondary solid tumors, particularly breast cancer.

- ESHL was first treated with extended-field, high-dose RT since early 1950s, with greater than 90% complete remission, but 30% relapse rates and long-term toxicity, including heart and lung damage, as well as secondary solid malignancies, such as breast, lung, and GI tract cancers.

- Mustargen, vincristine, procarbazine, and prednisone (MOPP) chemotherapy regimen was first published in 1970 and subsequently was shown to achieve long-term remissions in advanced disease by DeVita et al.[8]; doxorubicin, bleomycin, vinblastine, and dacarbazine (ABVD) was first reported and compared to MOPP by Bonadonna et al.[9] in 1975, also in advanced disease.

- Randomized study of MOPP vs. ABVD (both with mantle-field radiation) in ESHL showed improved relapse-free survival (RFS), similar OS, but decreased hematologic toxicity and infertility for the ABVD arm, making ABVD the standard initial chemotherapy regimen (EORTC H6U trial).[10]

- RT vs. CMT: CMT showed better freedom from treatment failure (FFTF).
  - Subtotal nodal radiation (STLI) was used alone or in combination with chemotherapy in two prospective randomized trials, with improved FFTF for the CMT arms in each of them (HD7 GHSG: 2-year FFTF 96% vs. 87%; Southwest Oncology Group: 3-year FFS 94% vs. 81%) but without a significant difference in OS.[11,12]
  - CMT with involved field radiation therapy (IFRT) vs. STLI still showed significantly better RFS rate than radiation alone (European Organization for Research and Treatment of Cancer (EORTC)/ Groupe d'Etude des Lymphomes de l'Adulte (GELA) H7F and H8F).[13,14]

- RT field reduction: CMT with extended-field radiation therapy (EFRT) is not necessary to maintain FFTF.

- The majority of patients have a large mediastinal mass (LMA) and are at unfavorable risk.
- An Italian study randomized 140 patients with ESHL (IA, bulky IB/IIA, and IIEA) to four cycles of ABVD followed by STLI or by IFRT. The RT dose was 30 Gy to uninvolved and 36 Gy to involved sites.
    - After a median follow-up of 116 months, CR rates were 100% after ABVD plus STLI vs. 97% after ABVD plus IFRT; 12-year FFTF was 93% vs. 94% and OS 96% vs. 94%, respectively.[15]
- The EORTC H8U trial randomly assigned unfavorable patients to MOPP/ABVD for four cycles followed by IFRT (36–40 Gy) or by STLI (same dose). FFTF was the same in both groups (92% in each arm).[16]
- The GHSG HD8 study randomly assigned unfavorable ESHL patients to receive four cycles of cyclophosphamide, vincristine, procarbazine, and prednisone (COPP)/ABVD followed by either extended or involved field RT.
    - At a median follow-up of 56 months, FFTF was 86% (in each arm) and no difference in relapse rate or survival was observed.
    - Acute side effects were more frequent in patients who received the extended field radiotherapy.[17]
- Reduction in the number of chemotherapy cycles and dose of RT may also be accomplished without loss of FFTF.
    - HD10 trial of the GHSG randomly assigned 1,370 patients with favorable ESHL to four cycles of ABVD plus 30 Gy IFRT (standard, arm A), four cycles of ABVD plus 20 Gy IFRT (arm B), two cycles of ABVD plus 30 Gy IFRT (arm C), or two cycles ABVD plus 20 Gy IFRT (arm D).
        - Of 847 patients evaluable at second interim analysis in August 2003 when the median observation time was 28 months, CR was 98%, only 1% of patients had either progressive disease or no change, and 2.5% had relapsed.
        - With overall OS of 99% and FFTF of 97%, there were no statistical differences in OS or FFTF between the four arms.

- The trend was toward increased relapse rate with 20 Gy IFRT.
- Due to short follow-up and few events, final judgement will be reserved until the results mature.[18]

- A similarly designed HD11 German trial for unfavorable ESHL randomized 1,570 patients to four groups treated with either four cycles of ABVD or BEACOPP (see advanced disease below) and with either 20 or 30 Gy IFRT.
  - As in HD10, the four arms were equivalent in CR (95–97%), FFTF (87–90% at 3 years), and OS (96–97% at 3 years), with slightly more relapses in 20 Gy arms (9% vs 6%).
  - BEACOPP and 30 Gy arms had higher toxicity, with increased secondary malignancy in BEACOPP arm despite short follow-up.
  - This leaves ABVD plus IFRT, likely 30 Gy, as standard.[19]

- Chemotherapy alone: likely more relapses, possibly lower OS than with CMT
  - At Memorial Sloan-Kettering Cancer Center, 152 patients with stages I-IIIA nonbulky disease were randomized to six cycles of ABVD alone or ABVD for six cycles and EFRT.
    - CR was 94% in both arms. At 5 years, there were no statistically significant differences in outcomes for CMT vs. ABVD alone: CR duration 91% vs. 87% ($P=.61$), FFTF 86% vs. 81% ($P=.6$), and OS 97% vs. 91% ($P=.08$).
    - Even though OS trend favors CMT, the study was not powered to detect benefits less than 20%, and no conclusion regarding the trend can be drawn.[20]
  - Nachman et al. for the Children's Cancer Group (CCG) randomly assigned 501 patients who achieved an initial CR to risk-adapted combination chemotherapy to low-dose IFRT (21 Gy) or no further treatment.
    - Patients receiving CMT had an OS of 92% vs. 87% for patients treated with chemotherapy alone ($P=.057$).

- However, if one analyzes the data by therapy received, there is a survival benefit for CMT ($P=.0024$).[21]
- An intergroup study (NCI of Canada and Eastern Cooperative Oncology Group) compared standard therapy STLI (favorable patients) or two cycles of ABVD and STLI (unfavorable patients) to four cycles of ABVD alone for both favorable and unfavorable patients.
  - The median duration of follow-up is 4.2 years. The experimental arm, four cycles of ABVD, had an inferior PFS to that of standard therapy ($P=.006$).[22]
- EORTC/GELA H9-F trial randomized 578 favorable early stage patients achieving CR/CRu after six cycles of EBVP (epirubicin, bleomycin, vinblastine, and prednisone) to either IFRT of 36 Gy, IFRT of 20 Gy, or to no radiation.
  - The arm without RT closed due to an excessive number of relapses.
  - After median follow-up of 51 months, 4-year event-free survival (EFS) rates were 88%, 85%, and 69%, and 4-year OS rates were 98%, 100%, and 98%, respectively.
    - Omission of RT thus resulted in inferior EFS ($P<.001$), whereas 20-Gy dose was equivalent to 36-Gy dose.[23]
- The evidence from these four studies suggests that for patients with ESHL without a large mediastinal mass four to six cycles of chemotherapy alone is inferior to the same chemotherapy and consolidative RT.

Treatment of Advanced Stage (IIB/III/IV) Disease (ASHL)

- This definition also includes stage II patients with LMA, extranodal disease, or massive splenic involvement.
- Landmark report by DeVita et al. in 1970 showed that MOPP achieved CR in over 80% of patients with ASHL and achieved long-term PFS in 50%.[24]
- The ABVD regimen pioneered by Bonadonna and colleagues[25] has replaced MOPP as the standard

chemotherapy program for HL, primarily due to a more favorable toxicity profile.

■ The modern era of ASHL treatment begins with the report by Canellos et al. of a randomized Cancer and Leukemia Group B (CALGB) trial of three regimens: six to eight cycles of ABVD, six to eight cycles of MOPP, and 12 cycles of MOPP alternating with ABVD, all without RT.

  * Patients relapsing with either MOPP or ABVD alone were switched to the opposite regimen.
  * The CR rate to MOPP was inferior to the other arms (67%, 82%, and 83% respectively; $P=.006$).
  * FFTF was also inferior with MOPP (50%, 61%, and 65%, respectively), but OS was the same in each arm, even at a median follow-up of 10 years.[26]
  * Similarity in OS reflected the ability of high-dose therapy and ASCT to salvage these patients.
  * Based on the equivalent efficacy of ABVD and MOPP alternating with ABVD, the better short- and long-term toxicity profile seen with ABVD alone makes ABVD the benchmark against which newer regimens need to be compared.

■ New regimens

  * MOPP/ABV hybrid consolidated MOPP and ABVD, omitted dacarbazine, and increased doxorubicin dose from 25 mg/m^2 to 35 mg/m^2.
    ■ Initial randomized studies showed superior FFS, but a randomized study of MOPP/ABV hybrid vs. ABVD for 8 to 10 cycles showed similar CR, FFS, and OS in 856 patients with median follow-up of 6 years.
    ■ MOPP/ABV hybrid was associated with increased acute hematologic and pulmonary toxicity as well as increased incidence of myelodysplastic syndrome (MDS)/acute myelogenous leukemia (AML).[27]
    ■ ABVD thus remained the standard.
  * From 1993–1998, the GHSG randomly assigned 1,201 patients with ASHL to eight cycles of COPP/ABVD (ABVD equivalent) to standard doses of BEACOPP (bleomycin, etoposide, doxorubicin, cyclophosphamide, vincristine, prednisone and procar-

bazine) or to escalated BEACOPP (increased etoposide, doxorubicin, cyclophosphamide doses).

- Patients received IFRT postchemotherapy if a residual nodal mass was at least 2 centimeters postchemotherapy or if there was bulky disease at presentation.
- At the first interim analysis, the COPP/ABVD arm was stopped due to inferior results.
- Two hundred and sixty patients received COPP/ABVD, 469 received BEACOPP, and 466 patients received escalated BEACOPP.
- At 5 years, FFTF and OS rates for COPP/ABVD, standard-dose BEACOPP, and escalated BEACOPP were 69% and 83%, 76% and 88%, and 87% and 91%, respectively.
- FFTF and OS were statistically significantly superior for escalated BEACOPP when compared to COPP/ABVD ($P=.04$ and $P=.002$, respectively).
- Escalated BEACOPP had higher incidence of grade 3/4 hematologic toxicity despite universal use of G-CSF.
- Five-year OS for patients with IPS of 0–3 are similar for COPP/ABVD, BEACOPP, and escalated BEACOPP: 84–92%, 86–93%, and 90–95%, respectively.
- The difference was significant in 5-year FFTF for patients with at least four IPS risk factors: 59% for COPP/ABVD, 74% for standard BEACOPP, and 82% for escalated BEACOPP (Figure 6-2).[28]
- Based on that trial, escalated BEACOPP may be considered standard therapy for patients with four or more IPI risk factors.
- HD12 trial with 1,593 patients comparing four cycles of BEACOPP followed by four cycles of regular BEACOPP to eight cycles of escalated BEACOPP, with or without RT, showed no significant differences in FFTF and OS at 2 years.[29]
- Recent data also show possibility of de-escalation to regular strength BEACOPP after negative interim PET scan.

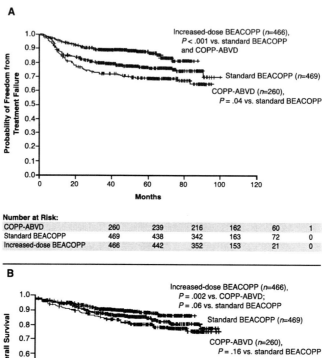

Number at Risk:

COPP-ABVD		260	239	216	162	60	1
Standard BEACOPP		469	438	342	163	72	0
Increased-dose BEACOPP		466	442	352	153	21	0

Number at Risk:

COPP-ABVD		260	239	216	162	60	1
Standard BEACOPP		469	438	342	163	72	0
Increased-dose BEACOPP		466	442	352	153	21	0

Figure 6-2: Kaplan–Meier analysis of the probability of freedom from treatment failure (Panel A) and overall survival (Panel B). *P* values were calculated with use of the log-rank test for all three pairwise differences between groups. Numbers in parentheses are the numbers of patients. COPP-ABVD denotes cyclophosphamide, vincristine, procarbazine, prednisone, doxorubicin, bleomycin, vinblastine, and dacarbazine and BEACOPP denotes bleomycin, etoposide, doxorubicin, cyclophosphamide, vincristine, procarbazine, and prednisone. Tick marks indicate censored survival data. Diehl et al. *NEJM* 348(24): 2386–2395, Figure 2, June 2003. Used with permission.

* Stanford V regimen is a short course of weekly chemotherapy for 12 weeks, with decreased cumulative doses of doxorubicin, nitrogen mustard, and bleomycin, with addition of etoposide and with more intensive consolidative radiotherapy.[30]
  * By definition, all lymph nodes greater than 5 cm pretreatment receive full-dose RT (36Gy).
  * Stanford had treated 142 patients with 5-year FFP of 89% and OS of 96%.
    * Patients with an IPS of 0–2 had a significantly superior FFP to those with scores of 3 or greater (94% vs. 75%, p= 0.0001).
    * There were no cases of secondary leukemia and 24 successful pregnancies.[31]
  * At Memorial Sloan-Kettering Cancer Center (MSKCC), 126 patients achieved 3-year FFTF of 80% and OS of 91% with a median follow-up of 36 months.[32]
    * Patients with 0–3 IPS factors had FFTF and OS of 86% and 95%, respectively. Patients with four or more factors had FFTF and OS of 50% and 75%, respectively.
    * Of 25 treatment failures, 14 were successfully salvaged with high-dose chemoradiotherapy and ASCT, for a 3-year freedom from second relapse of 55%.
    * No secondary leukemia was observed, and seven successful pregnancies were reported by 65 female patients.
  * The Italian Lymphoma Study group randomized 355 patients to ABVD, Stanford V, or a novel 10-drug regimen—MOPPEBVCAD.
    * Unlike in standard Stanford V, patients received RT only if they had bulky disease, and received it at median of 6 weeks after chemotherapy, not 2–4 weeks after.
    * With median follow-up of 61 months, Stanford V was inferior to ABVD and MOPPEBVCAD: CR rates were 76%, 89%, and 94%; 5-year FFS rates were 54%, 78%, and 81%; and 5-year OS rates were 82%, 90%, and 89%.[33]

- This randomized trial suggests that Stanford V depends on carefully administered radiotherapy for its efficacy and may be a valid treatment option for patients with ASHL that requires RT.
- A United States Intergroup trial comparing ABVD and Stanford V in ASHL is ongoing.

■ Upfront ASCT
- An intergroup study randomized poor risk patients to eight cycles of ABVD-equivalent chemotherapy or four cycles of the same chemotherapy followed by high-dose therapy and ASCT.
- There was no difference in the CR rate, FFS, or OS between the two arms.[34] Thus, upfront ASCT is not thought to be advantageous.

■ Consolidative RT: used as part of a planned CMT approach as with Stanford V or to convert an uncertain CR to a CR, as with escalated BEACOPP.
- The hypothesis is that radiation would improve FFTF by reducing relapse at bulky or residual disease sites. The results of initial randomized studies were conflicting.
- Loeffler et al. reported a meta-analysis of 14 randomized trials performed from 1972–1988 with data on 1,740 patients.
  - There were two distinct study designs: after initial chemotherapy, patients were randomized either to receive RT vs. observation or RT vs. additional chemotherapy.
  - In the additional RT-alone design, there was 11% improvement in CR duration in the RT groups ($P<.001$); OS was the same.
  - In contrast, when CMT was compared with the cohorts that received additional chemotherapy, CR duration was the same but OS was superior with patients who did not receive RT ($P=.045$).[35]
  - Nearly all the chemotherapy regimens used in these studies were MOPP or MOPP-equivalent regimens, which limits applicability of this meta-analysis, because such regimens are no longer used.

* Three recent randomized studies have added to the confusion.
  * GELA reported the results of a randomized study of 559 patients comparing two different chemo-therapy regimens (MOPP/ABV or ABVPP [doxorubicin, bleomycin, vinblastine, procarbazine and prednisone]) followed by a second randomization for patients achieving CR/partial remission (PR) to two more cycles of the same chemotherapy or STLI.
    * After induction chemotherapy, 418 patients were evaluated for the consolidation phase; the 5 year results have been recently updated at 10 years and appear consistent.
    * OS in the MOPP/ABV groups were the same between additional chemotherapy and RT (85% vs. 88% at 5 years; 78% vs. 82% at 10 years).
    * After ABVPP, OS was superior for the chemotherapy arm (94% vs. 78% at 5 years, $P = .002$; 90% vs. 77% at 10 years; $P = .03$).[36,37]
  * The CCG randomly assigned 501 patients achieving a CR to low-dose IFRT or observation.
    * The 3-year FFTF was 87% for all patients; 92% for those randomized to receive RT; and 87% randomized to observation ($P = .06$).
    * An alternative analysis based on therapy actually received excluded the patients randomized to receive RT who refused the intervention. In this "as treated" analysis, there was a significant improvement in FFTF for those patients who received RT (93% vs. 85%, $P = .002$).[38]
  * EORTC randomly assigned 421 patients in CR after MOPP/ABV chemotherapy to RT or observation.
    * The dose of RT was 24 Gy administered to all initially involved nodal sites and 16–24 Gy to all initially involved extranodal sites. Patients in PR were all treated with 30 Gy to nodal areas and 18–24 Gy to extranodal sites.
    * With median follow-up of 6.5 years, 5-year OS rates for the RT and observation groups were 85% and 91%, respectively ($P = .07$). Those

patients who had a partial response to MOPP/ABV had EFS and OS rates after RT of 79% and 87%.[39]

- Based on these three studies using ABVD-equivalent chemotherapy, RT clearly did not improve the outcome for patients in CR after full-course chemotherapy.

Treatment of Relapsed Disease

- Ten to 20% of patients have relapsed or primary refractory HL.
  - Ninety percent relapse within 2 years of initial treatment.
- Standard dose second-line chemotherapy (SDSC) results in low CR rates and minimal survival benefit.
  - Longo et al.[40] reported a median survival of only 16 months in 51 patients treated with MOPP chemotherapy who never achieved CR.
  - Similar results were seen in patients who failed MOPP/ABV hybrid or alternating regimens with a long-term EFS of 8%.[41]
- Multiple studies established that HDT with ASCT will induce long-term remissions in 40% of patients.
  - Two randomized studies comparing SDSC with HDT/ASCT were reported.
  - The British National Lymphoma Investigation (BNLI) randomly assigned relapsed and primary refractory patients to either BEAM HDT followed by ASCT or up to three cycles of mini-BEAM.[42]
  - The GHSG randomly assigned patients with relapsed HL to either two cycles of dexa-BEAM and BEAM and ASCT vs. four cycles of dexa-BEAM (Figure 6-3).[43]
  - Each study demonstrated a statistically significant improvement in both EFS and PFS for the patients treated on the HDT arms, but neither was powered to show an OS advantage.
- Transplant-related mortality decreased from 15% to less than 3% in most series with better supportive care and

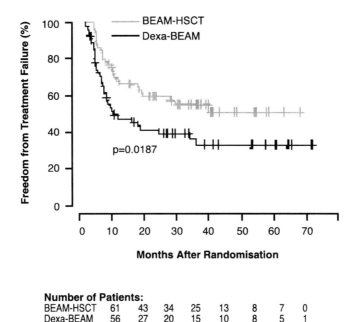

Number of Patients:

BEAM-HSCT	61	43	34	25	13	8	7	0
Dexa-BEAM	56	27	20	15	10	8	5	1

Figure 6-3: Freedom from treatment failure for patients with relapsed chemosensitive Hodgkin's disease. N. Schmitz et al; *Lancet* Volume 359, Issue 9323, 15 June 2002, Pages 2065–2071, Figure 3.

use of peripheral blood progenitor cells as opposed to bone marrow as the stem cell graft.

- Pretransplant cytoreduction with SDSC:
  - At MSKCC, 156 patients received treatment utilizing accelerated fractionation radiotherapy either as total lymphoid irradiation or as an IFRT followed by HDT and bone marrow infusion.
  - RT was incorporated into the program on the premise that just like with frontlike treatment, relapsed post HDT/ASCT would occur at the sites of initial nodal involvement.
  - At a median follow-up of 11 years, the EFS is 45% with no relapses occurring later than 36 months post-transplant.
  - After the introduction of G-CSF, overall mortality of the program decreased from 18% to 6%.

- Patients with chemosensitive disease to SDSC had a marked improvement in EFS compared to patients with refractory disease at the time of HDT. Chemosensitivity is now a requirement to proceed with HDT/ASCT.[44]
- Optimal SDSC regimen is unclear, but should result in adequate cytoreduction in at least 75% of patients without extramedullary toxicity or severe BM suppression with subsequent inability to collect an adequate stem cell harvest.
  - Moskowitz and colleagues reported a comprehensive program for the treatment of 82 patients with relapsed and primary refractory HL using SDSC containing ifosfamide, carboplatin, and etoposide (ICE); only responders were subsequently offered HDT and ASCT.
  - The response rate to ICE was 90% with no ICE related extramedullary toxicity and median number of CD34-positive cells collected was 7×10^6/kg (5×10^6/kg is considered sufficient for ASCT).
  - With median follow-up of 6 years, 55% of the patients remain alive and event free by intention-to-treat analysis.
  - In the subset of patients who received HDT/ASCT (75 of 82 patients), the EFS is 61%.[45]
  - Other SDSC regimens include DHAP (dexamethasone, high dose cytarabine, cisplatin), ESHAP (etoposide, methylprednisolone, high-dose cytarabine, cisplatin), and ASHAP (doxorubicin, methylprednisolone, high-dose cytarabine, cisplatin).
- Data conflict as to whether patients with primary refractory disease have worse outcomes with ASCT than patients with relapsed disease, partially because the definition of primary refractory disease differs among groups.
  - MSKCC transplanted 75 patients with primary refractory HL with a median follow-up of 10 years.
  - No difference in EFS for patients with chemosensitive primary refractory vs. chemosensitive relapsed disease.[46]

- HDT/ASCT should be considered as standard treatment for patients with primary refractory HD if chemosensitivity to SDSC is established.
- In addition to chemosensitivity to SDSC, other factors may be important in predicting survival.
  - In MSKCC study of ICE/HDT/ASCT extranodal sites of disease, initial response duration of less than 1 year and B symptoms at relapse predicted survival. [45]
  - A favorable risk group having zero or one of these risk factors (62% of the patients) had EFS of 83% measured from initiation of ICE therapy.
  - Patients with two or three risk factors faired less well, with EFSs of 27% and 10%, respectively.
  - Based on this three-factor model, a new trial was run:
    - Patients with zero or one risk factor received same therapy as before.
    - Patients with two risk factors received one dose of standard dose ICE followed by a dose of augmented ICE second-line therapy as well as a more dose intense transplant-conditioning regimen.
    - Patients with three risk factors received cytoreduction with two transplant doses of ICE each followed by stem cell support.
    - Patients had to have chemosensitive disease to initial "ICE."
    - With median follow-up of 32 months, patients with multiple risk factors have improved EFS for patients with 2–3 risk factors from 27% to 45% ($P=.07$), as compared to prior treatment without risk stratification.[47]
- Allogeneic stem cell transplantation (allo-SCT) should be used conservatively.
  - The advantages of allo-SCT is graft vs. lymphoma (GVL) effect and infusion of a lymphoma-free stem cell product.
    - Existence of graft vs. HL is likely but not proven.
    - Clinical evidence for GVL was seen in a study of reduced intensity allo-SCT where 16 of 49 patients with HL received donor lymphocyte infusion and 56% of them had CR/PR.[48]

- The disadvantage is high treatment-related mortality (TRM) compared to ASCT.
  - The European Group for Blood & Marrow Transplantation (EBMT) registry analysis of 1,185 lymphoma patients undergoing allo-SCT between 1982 and 1998 included 167 patients with HL.
  - TRM was extremely high at 51.7%.
  - HL was the only lymphoma that showed an inferior RFS as compared to ASCT.[49]
- Allo-SCT with reduced intensity (RIC) and nonmyeloablative (NMC) conditioning:
  - This approach relies primarily on GVL effect and not on cytoreduction provided by the conditioning regimens in an attempt to reduce TRM.
  - EBMT comparison of 99 patients receiving NMC and 154 patients receiving classical conditioning showed lower TRM for NMC group and higher OS, but both groups had relapse rates around 50% at 4 years.[50]
    - Chemoresistant disease prior to any allo-SCT predicted poor outcome.
  - BNLI examined 72 patients who failed ASCT, comparing 38 patients undergoing NMC allo-SCT with 34 matched eligible patients who received chemotherapy with or without RT.
    - NMC group had better actuarial 10-year OS of 48% vs. 15% for standard salvage therapy group.[51]
- NMC allo-SCT, but not conventional allo-SCT, is an option for those who failed ASCT and then demonstrated chemosensitive disease.
- Standard salvage therapy options (for patients not eligible for ASCT):
  - RT alone: rarely used
    - Review of GHSG database of 4,754 patients identified 100 patients salvaged with RT alone, most with ESHL.
    - CR was 77%, 5-year OS was 51%, and freedom from second failure (FF2F) was 28%, with median follow-up of 6 years.
    - Limited-stage disease and lack of B symptoms were favorable for OS and good performance status was favorable for FF2F.

- Low FF2F and better OS reflects the fact that RT is poor salvage therapy and OS is improved by subsequent treatment, which in this series was mostly conventional chemotherapy and HDT/ASCT.[52]
- Conventional chemotherapy: use a first-line therapy that was not given initially.
  - For most patients, initial therapy was ABVD, so remaining first-line therapies would be variants of MOPP, BEACOPP, and Stanford V.
  - Other salvage regimens include MINE (mitoguazone, ifosfamide, vinorelbine, etoposide), EVA (etoposide, vinblastine, doxorubicin), GND (gemcitabine, vinorelbine, liposomal doxorubicin), and many others.
  - Following salvage therapy, patients with CR1 of less than 12 months, B symptoms, and advanced stage at relapse have worse outcomes.
    - Note that these factors are similar to the three risk factors for outcomes after HDT/ASCT.
  - Long-term remissions are uncommon.

Long-Term Toxicity: Secondary Cancer (SC) and Cardiovascular Disease (CVD)

- After 10–15 years post treatment, the risk of long-term toxicity exceeds the rate of HL recurrence.
- Aleman et al. reviewed 1,261 patients treated for HL with median follow-up of 18 years, of which 534 died, 55% from HL.
  - Relative risks (RR) of dying from solid tumors was 6.6 and from CVD 6.3 as compared to general population.[53]
- British cohort of 5,519 patients treated from 1963–1993 noted 322 SC.
  - In this study, breast cancer increase was relatively low (RR 2.5) and was associated with RT before the age of 25 (RR 14.4).
  - GI cancer risk had RR of 3.4 after CMT, increasing to 18.7 with CMT before age 25.
  - Lung cancer risk increased more with CMT (RR 4.3) than with either modality alone.

- Leukemia risk increased with chemotherapy (RR 31.6) and CMT (RR 38.1) and was greater with chemotherapy before age 25 (RR 85.2).[54]
- Breast cancer: younger age and higher RT dose via mantle field increase the risk.
    - Travis et al. evaluated 3,817 women diagnosed before the age of 30 between 1965 and 1994, with a mean dose of radiation delivered to the breast of 25.1 Gy.
        - Breast cancer developed in 105 patients at mean of 18 years post-therapy; cases were matched to 266 patients with HL without breast cancer.
        - RT alone had RR of 3.2, decreasing to 1.4 with CMT, compared to decreased risk with alkylator-based chemotherapy alone (RR 0.6), likely due to premature menopause.
        - RT over 4 Gy to the breast increased RR to 3.2 and over 40 Gy to 8.0.[55]
        - Risk did not vary by age in this study of women all under the age of 30; other studies that examined wider age intervals noted the impact of age.
            - van Leeuwen et al. analyzed data on 1,253 adolescent and young adult patients treated between 1966 and 1986 with mean follow-up of 14.1 years.
            - Relative risk of all SC was higher for younger patients: for breast cancer, RR was 16.9 for patients younger than 20 years old, 5.6 for those aged 21–30, and 2.4 for those aged 31–39 (Figure 6.4).[56]
    - As a result of increased breast cancer risk, the use of mantle-field RT should be minimized for women younger than 30.
    - Modern RT has much smaller fields and smaller RT doses in 20–36 Gy range.
- Other solid tumors
    - Lung cancer contributes the most to excess mortality, smoking after RT increases the risk.
    - GI cancers are probably second major contributor to excess mortality; risks with CMT are greater than RT, and risks with RT are greater than chemotherapy alone.

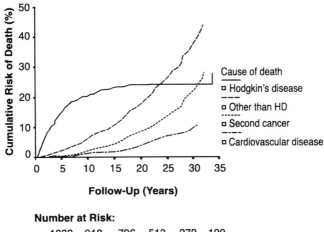

Figure 6-4: The actuarial risks of death from major disease categories. HD, Hodgkin's disease. BMP Aleman et al: *J Clin Oncol* 21;2003:3431–3439. Figure 1. Used with permission from ASCO.

- Bone and soft tissue cancer is likely more RT related.
- Thyroid cancer is RT related, and the risk is more prominent in children.
- Melanoma RR is about 2; risk factors are unclear.
- MDS/AML
    - Incidence low at 1–3%, but greatly increased compared to general population, as noted above.
    - Most are alkylator related (chromosome 5 and 7 losses), and thus are seen 5–10 years from treatment.
    - ABVD has decreased leukemogenic potential as compared with alkylator-based regimens (MOPP), so the risk is lower and is related more to topoisomerase II inhibitors such as doxorubicin and etoposide (11q23 translocations seen within first 2–3 years of treatment).
- NHL: incidence 1–1.5%, usually DLBCL; risk factors unclear and may be related to HL itself.
- CVD:
    - Hancock et al. examined the outcomes of 2,232 patients treated between 1960 and 1991, with a median follow-up of 9.5 years.

- 3.9% died of heart disease; 55 of those 88 died from myocardial infarction (MI).
- Mediastinal RT over 30 Gy had RR of 3.5 for cardiac death, with risk highest for RT before the age of 20.
- Blocking to limit cardiac exposure did not decrease the risk from MI.[57]
- Maintain a high index of suspicion for MI in patients in their 30s and 40s with chest pain who received mantle-field RT.
- Anthracycline cardiotoxicity likely contributes to cardiac mortality.
- Bleomycin pulmonary toxicity:
  - Highest in patients over 40 years old
  - Lowered 5-year OS from 90% to 63% in one series[58]
  - Omission of bleomycin did not impact PFS or OS.
  - An ongoing Cancer and Leukemia Group B trial attempts to eliminate bleomycin and dacarbazine and bring in gemcitabine front-line in a randomized assignment to ABVD or AVG.

■ General Treatment Approach

- Early stage (ESHL):
  - Very favorable ESHL: IFRT.
  - Favorable ESHL: CMT with two to four cycles of ABVD followed by 20–36 Gy IFRT
  - Unfavorable ESHL: CMT with four cycles of ABVD followed by 30–36 Gy IFRT
  - These recommendations must be made with caution in light of the increased incidence of secondary breast cancer in young women treated with CMT.
- Advanced stage (ASHL):
  - IPS 0–3, nonbulky: six cycles of ABVD
  - IPS 0–3, bulky: six cycles of ABVD plus 30–36 Gy IFRT *or* Stanford V (includes IFRT)
  - IPS 4–7: eight cycles of escalated BEACOPP (includes IFRT)
- Relapsed/refractory disease:
  - ASCT candidate: preparative second-line chemotherapy (ICE, DHAP, ESHAP, or ASHAP):

- If sensitive to second-line therapy, proceed with HDT/ASCT.
- If resistant, palliative chemotherapy (another salvage regimen such as MINE, EVA, GND, or single-agent vinorelbine)
  - Not an ASCT candidate:
    - Second-line chemotherapy with non-cross-resistant regimen (for initial ABVD therapy this would be MOPP, BEACOPP, or Stanford V), or
    - Another salvage regimen (such as MINE, EVA, GND)
  - Relapse after ASCT: second-line chemotherapy as above: if sensitive, consider NMC allo-SCT

■ Nodular Lymphocyte Predominant Hodgkin's Lymphoma (NLPHL)

Epidemiology/Presentation

- Five percent of all HL, median age mid-30s with wide distribution, male to female ratio skewed 3:1 or more
- Slightly higher risk of developing NHL at 2–5% than in cHL, with transformation to DLBCL showing clonal relationship
- Greater tendency for late relapse than cHL (overall relapse rates similar); relapses may be multiple
- Painless peripheral lymphadenopathy that spares mediastinum
- Over 80% present with early stage disease.

Pathology

Morphology

- Typical neoplastic cells are L&H HRS variant cells that are called "popcorn" cell for the bulging nuclear lobes.
- Nodular pattern with few inflammatory cells such as neutrophils, eosinophils, or plasma cells that are often seen in cHL.
- Significant follicular dendritic cell (FDC) meshwork within nodules.

- Lymphocytes and histiocytes may be present in the background.
- Nodules may be interrupted by small aggregates of T cells.
- May be difficult to distinguish from T-cell/histiocyte-rich subtype of diffuse large B-cell lymphoma (T/HRBCL) Review of 218 cases showed a difference in reactive cellular background:[59]
  - NLPHL background had more small B cells and CD3+CD4+CD57+ T cells, while background cells in T/HRBCL mostly consisted of CD8+ cytotoxic T cells and histiocytes.
  - HLPHL had expanded meshworks of FDCs, while T/HRBCL did not.

Immunophenotype

- L&H cells express B-cell antigens and CD45, but not CD30 or CD15, unlike in cHL.
- Bcl-6 positive, EMA negative; unlike cHL, usually EBV negative.

Cytogenetic and Molecular Changes

- In most cases of NLPHL, the rearranged Ig genes carry no crippling mutation. In fact, there is evidence of ongoing somatic mutations.[60]
- In contrast to cHL, the LPHL tumor clone shows evidence of selection for expression of a functional antigen receptor. This is supported by the detection of mRNA for kappa or lambda light chains in the HRS cells in NLPHL, but not cHL.
- Chromosomal number abnormalities as in cHL

Treatment

- Excellent prognosis; 90% CR and over 90% 10-year OS
- Most cases were reclassified from cHL post-treatment and were thus treated like early stage cHL with similar excellent outcomes; thus there are very few studies of treatment tailored to NLPHL.

▪ If diagnosed de novo, they may likely be treated with IFRT for localized disease and with treatments similar to classical HL for advanced or unfavorable localized disease.

▪ Single-agent rituximab results in 90-100% ORR in 2 phase II trials but remains experimental.
  ◦ Stanford study showed short median freedom from progression of only 10.2 months.[61]
  ◦ A German study, on the other side, showed a median time to progression of 31 months.[62]

Progressive Transformation of Follicular Centers (PTGC)

▪ A type of follicular lymphoid hyperplasia that carries a lifetime risk of developing NLPHL of about 20%; conversely, 20% of NLPHL will also have evidence of PTGC.

■ References

1. Hjalgrim H, Askling J, Rostgaard K, et al. Characteristics of Hodgkin's lymphoma after infectious mononucleosis. *N Engl J Med*. 2003;349(14):1324–1332.

2. Vassilakopoulos TP, Angelopoulou MK, Constantinou N, et al. Development and validation of a clinical prediction rule for bone marrow involvement in patients with Hodgkin lymphoma. *Blood*. 2005;105(5):1875–1880.

3. Hutchings M, Loft A, Hansen M, et al. FDG-PET after two cycles of chemotherapy predicts treatment failure and progression-free survival in Hodgkin lymphoma. *Blood*. 2006; 107(1):52–59.

4. Diehl V, Harris NL, Mauch PM. Section 5: Hodgkin's Lymphoma. In: DeVita VT, Hellman S, Rosenberg SA, eds. *Cancer: Principles & Practice of Oncology*. Philadelphia: Lippincott Williams & Wilkins; 2005:2020–2075.

5. Kuppers R, Rajewsky K, Zhao M, et al. Hodgkin disease: Hodgkin and Reed-Sternberg cells picked from histological sections show clonal immunoglobulin gene rearrangements and appear to be derived from B cells at various stages of development. *Proc Natl Acad Sci USA*. 1994;91(23): 10962–10966.

6.   Marafioti T, Hummel M, Anagnostopoulos I, et al. Origin of nodular lymphocyte-predominant Hodgkin's disease from a clonal expansion of highly mutated germinal-center B cells. *N Engl J Med.* 1997;337(7):453–458.

7.   Hasenclever D, Diehl V. A prognostic score for advanced Hodgkin's disease. International Prognostic Factors Project on Advanced Hodgkin's Disease. *N Engl J Med.* 1998; 339(21):1506–1514.

8.   Devita VT, Jr., Serpick AA, Carbone PP. Combination chemotherapy in the treatment of advanced Hodgkin's disease. *Ann Intern Med.* 1970;73(6):881–895.

9.   Bonadonna G, Zucali R, Monfardini S, De Lena M, Uslenghi C. Combination chemotherapy of Hodgkin's disease with adriamycin, bleomycin, vinblastine, and imidazole carboxamide versus MOPP. *Cancer.* 1975;36(1):252–259.

10.   Carde P, Hagenbeek A, Hayat M, et al. Clinical staging versus laparotomy and combined modality with MOPP versus ABVD in early-stage Hodgkin's disease: the H6 twin randomized trials from the European Organization for Research and Treatment of Cancer Lymphoma Cooperative Group. *J Clin Oncol.* 1993;11(11):2258–2272.

11.   Sieber M, Franklin J, Tesch H, et al. Two cycles of ABVD plus extended field radiotherapy is superior to radiotherapy alone in early stage Hodgkin's disease: Results of the German Hodgkin's Lymphoma Study Group (GHSG) trial HD7. *Blood.* 2002;100:341a.

12.   Press OW, LeBlanc M, Lichter AS, et al. Phase III randomized intergroup trial of subtotal lymphoid irradiation versus doxorubicin, vinblastine, and subtotal lymphoid irradiation for stage IA to IIA Hodgkin's disease. *J Clin Oncol.* 2001;19(22):4238–4244.

13.   Noordijk EM, Carde P, Dupouy N, et al. Combined-modality therapy for clinical stage I or II Hodgkin's lymphoma: long-term results of the European Organisation for Research and Treatment of Cancer H7 randomized controlled trials. *J Clin Oncol.* 2006;24(19):3128–3135.

14.   Hagenbeek A, Eghbali H, Ferme C, et al. Three cycles of MOPP/ABV (M/A) hybrid and involved-field irradiation is more effective than subtotal nodal irradiation (STNI) in favorable supradiaphragmatic clinical stages (CS) I-I Hodgkin's disease (HD): preliminary results of the EORTC-GELA H8-F randomized trial in 543 patients. *Blood.* 2000;96:575a.

15. Bonadonna G, Bonfante V, Viviani S, Di Russo A, Villani F, Valagussa P. ABVD plus subtotal nodal versus involved-field radiotherapy in early-stage Hodgkin's disease: long-term results. *J Clin Oncol*. 2004;22(14):2835–2841.

16. Fermé C, Eghbali H, Hagenbeek A, et al. MOPP/ABV hybrid and irradiation in unfavorable supradiaphragmatic clinical stages I-II Hodgkin s disease: Comparison of three treatment modalities. Preliminary results of the EORTC-GELA H8-U randomized trial in 995 patients. *Blood*. 2000;96:576a.

17. Engert A, Schiller P, Josting A, et al. Involved-field radiotherapy is equally effective and less toxic compared with extended-field radiotherapy after four cycles of chemotherapy in patients with early-stage unfavorable Hodgkin's lymphoma: results of the HD8 trial of the German Hodgkin's Lymphoma Study Group. *J Clin Oncol*. 2003;21(19): 3601–3608.

18. Engert A, Pluetschow A, Eich H, et al. Combined modality treatment of two or four cycles of ABVD followed by involved field radiotherapy in the treatment of patients with early stage Hodgkin's lymphoma: update interim analysis of the randomised HD10 study of the German Hodgkin Study Group. *Blood*. 2005;106(11):2673a.

19. Diehl V, Brillant C, Engert A, et al. Recent Interim Analysis of the HD11 Trial of the GHSG: Intensification of Chemotherapy and Reduction of Radiation Dose in Early Unfavorable Stage Hodgkin's Lymphoma. *Blood*. 2005; 106(11):816a.

20. Straus DJ, Portlock CS, Qin J, et al. Results of a prospective randomized clinical trial of doxorubicin, bleomycin, vinblastine, and dacarbazine (ABVD) followed by radiation therapy (RT) versus ABVD alone for stages I, II, and IIIA nonbulky Hodgkin disease. *Blood*. 2004;104(12):3483–3489.

21. Nachman JB, Sposto R, Herzog P, et al. Randomized comparison of low-dose involved-field radiotherapy and no radiotherapy for children with Hodgkin's disease who achieve a complete response to chemotherapy. *J Clin Oncol*. 2002; 20(18):3765–3771.

22. Meyer RM, Gospodarowicz MK, Connors JM, et al. Randomized comparison of ABVD chemotherapy with a strategy that includes radiation therapy in patients with limited-stage Hodgkin's lymphoma: National Cancer Institute of Canada Clinical Trials Group and the Eastern

Cooperative Oncology Group. *J Clin Oncol.* 2005;23(21): 4634–4642.

23.   Eghbali H, Brice P, Creemers G-Y, et al. Comparison of Three Radiation Dose Levels after EBVP Regimen in Favorable Supradiaphragmatic Clinical Stages (CS) I-II Hodgkin's Lymphoma (HL): Preliminary Results of the EORTC-GELA H9-F Trial. *Blood.* 2005;106(11):814a.

24.   Longo DL, Young RC, Wesley M, et al. Twenty years of MOPP therapy for Hodgkin's disease. *J Clin Oncol.* 1986; 4(9):1295–1306.

25.   Bonadonna G, Santoro A. ABVD chemotherapy in the treatment of Hodgkin's disease. *Cancer Treatment Reviews.* 1982; 9(1):21–35.

26.   Canellos GP, Anderson JR, Propert KJ, et al. Chemotherapy of advanced Hodgkin's disease with MOPP, ABVD, or MOPP alternating with ABVD. *N Engl J Med.* 1992; 327(21):1478–1484.

27.   Duggan DB, Petroni GR, Johnson JL, et al. Randomized comparison of ABVD and MOPP/ABV hybrid for the treatment of advanced Hodgkin's disease: report of an intergroup trial. *J Clin Oncol.* 2003;21(4):607–614.

28.   Diehl V, Franklin J, Pfreundschuh M, et al. Standard and increased-dose BEACOPP chemotherapy compared with COPP-ABVD for advanced Hodgkin's disease. *N Engl J Med.* 2003;348(24):2386–2395.

29.   Engert A, Franklin J, Mueller RP, et al. HD12 Randomised Trial Comparing 8 Dose-Escalated Cycles of BEACOPP with 4 Escalated and 4 Baseline Cycles in Patients with Advanced Stage Hodgkin Lymphoma (HL): An Analysis of the German Hodgkin Lymphoma Study Group (GHSG), University of Cologne, D-50924 Cologne, Germany. *Blood.* 2006;108(11):99a.

30.   Bartlett NL, Rosenberg SA, Hoppe RT, Hancock SL, Horning SJ. Brief chemotherapy, Stanford V, and adjuvant radiotherapy for bulky or advanced-stage Hodgkin's disease: a preliminary report. *J Clin Oncol.* 1995;13(5):1080–1088.

31.   Horning SJ, Hoppe RT, Breslin S, Bartlett NL, Brown BW, Rosenberg SA. Stanford V and radiotherapy for locally extensive and advanced Hodgkin's disease: mature results of a prospective clinical trial. *J Clin Oncol.* 2002;20(3): 630–637.

32.   Yahalom J, Edwards-Bennet S, Jacobs J, et al. Stanford V and Radiotherapy for Advanced and Locally Extensive

Hodgkins Disease (HD): The Memorial Sloan-Kettering Cancer Center (MSKCC) Experience. *Blood.* 2003; 102(12):1459a.

33.   Gobbi PG, Levis A, Chisesi T, et al. ABVD versus modified stanford V versus MOPPEBVCAD with optional and limited radiotherapy in intermediate- and advanced-stage Hodgkin's lymphoma: final results of a multicenter randomized trial by the Intergruppo Italiano Linfomi. *J Clin Oncol.* 2005;23(36):9198–9207.

34.   Federico M, Bellei M, Brice P, et al. High-dose therapy and autologous stem-cell transplantation versus conventional therapy for patients with advanced Hodgkin's lymphoma responding to front-line therapy. *J Clin Oncol.* 2003;21(12): 2320–2325.

35.   Loeffler M, Brosteanu O, Hasenclever D, et al. Meta-analysis of chemotherapy versus combined modality treatment trials in Hodgkin's disease. International Database on Hodgkin's Disease Overview Study Group. *J Clin Oncol.* 1998;16(3):818–829.

36.   Ferme C, Sebban C, Hennequin C, et al. Comparison of chemotherapy to radiotherapy as consolidation of complete or good partial response after six cycles of chemotherapy for patients with advanced Hodgkin's disease: results of the groupe d'etudes des lymphomes de l'Adulte H89 trial. *Blood.* 2000;95(7):2246–2252.

37.   Ferme C, Mounier N, Casasnovas O, et al. Long-term results and competing risk analysis of the H89 trial in patients with advanced-stage Hodgkin lymphoma: a study by the Groupe d'Etude des Lymphomes de l'Adulte (GELA). *Blood.* 2006;107(12):4636–4642.

38.   Nachman JB, Sposto R, Herzog P, et al. Randomized comparison of low-dose involved-field radiotherapy and no radiotherapy for children with Hodgkin's disease who achieve a complete response to chemotherapy. *J Clin Oncol.* 2002; 20(18):3765–3771.

39.   Aleman BM, Raemaekers JM, Tirelli U, et al. Involved-field radiotherapy for advanced Hodgkin's lymphoma. *N Engl J Med.* 2003;348(24):2396–2406.

40.   Longo DL, Duffey PL, Young RC, et al. Conventional-dose salvage combination chemotherapy in patients relapsing with Hodgkin's disease after combination chemotherapy: the low probability for cure. *J Clin Oncol.* 1992;10(2): 210–218.

41. Bonfante V, Santoro A, Viviani S, et al. Outcome of patients with Hodgkin's disease failing after primary MOPP-ABVD. *J Clin Oncol.* 1997;15(2):528–534.

42. Linch DC, Winfield D, Goldstone AH, et al. Dose intensification with autologous bone-marrow transplantation in relapsed and resistant Hodgkin's disease: results of a BNLI randomised trial. *Lancet.* 1993;341(8852):1051–1054.

43. Schmitz N, Pfistner B, Sextro M, et al. Aggressive conventional chemotherapy compared with high-dose chemotherapy with autologous haemopoietic stem-cell transplantation for relapsed chemosensitive Hodgkin's disease: a randomised trial. *Lancet.* 2002;359(9323):2065–2071.

44. Yahalom J, Gulati SC, Toia M, et al. Accelerated hyperfractionated total-lymphoid irradiation, high-dose chemotherapy, and autologous bone marrow transplantation for refractory and relapsing patients with Hodgkin's disease. *J Clin Oncol.* 1993;11(6):1062–1070.

45. Moskowitz CH, Nimer SD, Zelenetz AD, et al. A two-step comprehensive high-dose chemoradiotherapy second-line program for relapsed and refractory Hodgkin disease: analysis by intent to treat and development of a prognostic model. *Blood.* 2001;97(3):616–623.

46. Moskowitz CH, Kewalramani T, Nimer SD, Gonzalez M, Zelenetz AD, Yahalom J. Effectiveness of high dose chemoradiotherapy and autologous stem cell transplantation for patients with biopsy-proven primary refractory Hodgkin's disease. *Br J Haematol.* 2004;124(5):645–652.

47. Moskowitz CH, Kewalramani T, Nimer SD, et al. Risk-Adapted High Dose Chemoradiotherapy and ASCT for Patients with Relapsed and Primary Refractory Hodgkins Disease: An Intent to Treat Analysis. *Blood.* 2003; 102(11):403a.

48. Peggs KS, Hunter A, Chopra R, et al. Clinical evidence of a graft-versus-Hodgkin's-lymphoma effect after reduced-intensity allogeneic transplantation. *Lancet.* 2005;365(9475): 1934–1941.

49. Peniket AJ, Ruiz de Elvira MC, Taghipour G, et al. An EBMT registry matched study of allogeneic stem cell transplants for lymphoma: allogeneic transplantation is associated with a lower relapse rate but a higher procedure-related mortality rate than autologous transplantation. *Bone Marrow Transplantation.* 2003;31(8):667–678.

50. Sureda A, Robinson S, de Elvira CR, et al. Non Myeloablative Allogeneic Stem Cell Transplantation Significantly

Reduces Transplant Related Mortality in Comparison with Conventional Allogeneic Transplantation in Relapsed or Refractory Hodgkins Disease: Results of the European Group for Blood and Marrow Transplantation. *Blood.* 2003; 102(11):692a.

51. Thomson KJ, Peggs KS, Smith P, et al. Improved Outcome Following Reduced Intensity Allogeneic Transplantation in Hodgkin's Lymphoma Relapsing Post-Autologous Transplantation. *Blood.* 2005;106(11):657a.

52. Josting A, Nogova L, Franklin J, et al. Salvage radiotherapy in patients with relapsed and refractory Hodgkin's lymphoma: a retrospective analysis from the German Hodgkin Lymphoma Study Group. *J Clin Oncol.* 2005;23(7):1522–1529.

53. Aleman BM, van den Belt-Dusebout AW, Klokman WJ, et al. Long-term cause-specific mortality of patients treated for Hodgkin's disease. *J Clin Oncol.* 2003;21(18):3431–3439.

54. Swerdlow AJ, Barber JA, Hudson GV, et al. Risk of second malignancy after Hodgkin's disease in a collaborative British cohort: the relation to age at treatment. *J Clin Oncol.* 2000;18(3):498–509.

55. Travis LB, Hill DA, Dores GM, et al. Breast cancer following radiotherapy and chemotherapy among young women with Hodgkin disease. *JAMA.* 2003;290(4):465–475.

56. van Leeuwen FE, Klokman WJ, Veer MB, et al. Long-term risk of second malignancy in survivors of Hodgkin's disease treated during adolescence or young adulthood. *J Clin Oncol.* 2000;18(3):487–497.

57. Hancock SL, Tucker MA, Hoppe RT. Factors affecting late mortality from heart disease after treatment of Hodgkin's disease. *JAMA.* 1993;270(16):1949–1955.

58. Martin WG, Ristow KM, Habermann TM, et al. Bleomycin pulmonary toxicity has a negative impact on the outcome of patients with Hodgkin's lymphoma. *J Clin Oncol.* 2005; 23(30):7614–7620.

59. Boudova L, Torlakovic E, Delabie J, et al. Nodular lymphocyte-predominant Hodgkin lymphoma with nodules resembling T-cell/histiocyte-rich B-cell lymphoma: differential diagnosis between nodular lymphocyte-predominant Hodgkin lymphoma and T-cell/histiocyte-rich B-cell lymphoma. *Blood.* 2003;102(10):3753–3758.

60. Chan WC. Cellular origin of nodular lymphocyte-predominant Hodgkin's lymphoma: immunophenotypic and molecular studies. *Seminars in Hematology.* 1999;36(3):242–252.

61. Ekstrand BC, Lucas JB, Horwitz SM, et al. Rituximab in lymphocyte-predominant Hodgkin disease: results of a phase 2 trial. *Blood*. 2003;101(11):4285–4289.

62. Schulz H, Trelle S, Reiser M, Sieber M, Diehl V, Engert A. Rituximab in Relapsed Lymphocyte Predominant Hodgkin's Disease (LPHD). Long-Term Results of a Phase-II Study from the German Hodgkin Lymphoma Study Group (GHSG). *Blood*. 2005;106(11):1503a.

Chemotherapy Regimens

Abbreviations: AUC, area under curve; IT, intrathecal; IV, intravenous; IVCI, IV continuous infusion; IVP, IV push; IVPB, IV piggyback; PO, oral; SC, subcutaneous.

■ Hodgkin's Lymphoma

Initial Treatment, Early Stage

ABVD: *Every 2 weeks (2 doses equals 1 cycle)*

Agent	Dose	Days
Adriamycin (doxorubicin)	25 mg/m^2 IVP	1 and 15
Bleomycin	10 U/m^2 IV	1 and 15
Vinblastine	6 mg/m^2 IVP	1 and 15
Dacarbazine	375 mg/m^2 IVPB	1 and 15

MOPP: *Every 3 weeks.*

Agent	Dose	Days
Mechlorethamine	6 mg/m^2 IVP	1 and 8
Oncovin (vincristine)	1.4 mg/m^2 IVP (2 mg cap)	1 and 8
Procarbazine	100 mg/m^2 PO	1–14

■ Note

■ COPP uses cyclophosphamide 650 mg/m^2 instead of mechlorethamine.

■ Reference

Canellos GP, Anderson JR, Propert KJ, et al. Chemotherapy of advanced Hodgkin's disease with MOPP, ABVD, or MOPP alternating with ABVD. *N Engl J Med.* 1992;327(21):1478–1484.

Initial Treatment, Advanced Stage (in addition to ABVD)

Stanford V: *Three cycles of 4 weekly treatments (12 weeks total) followed in 2–4 weeks by 36 by IFRT (for disease greater than 5 cm or splenic involvement).*

Agent	Dose	Days
Doxorubicin	25 mg/m^2 IVP	1 and 15
Vinblastine	6 mg/m^2 IVP	1 and 15
Mechlorethamine	6 mg/m^2 IV	1
Etoposide	60 mg/m^2 IVPB	15
Etoposide	120 mg/m^2 PO	16
Vincristine	1.4 mg/m^2 IVP (2 mg cap)	8 and 22
Bleomycin	5 U/m^2 IV	8 and 22
Prednisone	40 mg/m^2 PO	Every other day*

■ Notes

■ *Taper prednisone by 10 mg every other day during weeks 11 and 12.

■ For patients older than 50 years, starting with the third cycle reduce vinblastine to 4 mg/m^2 and vincristine to 1 mg/m^2.

■ If ANC is less than 1,000, reduce doses of doxorubicin, vinblastine, mechlorethamine, and etoposide (myelosuppressive drugs) by 35%; if ANC is less than 500, delay treatment for 1 week (no delays for other, nonmyelosuppressive drugs).

- If dose reduction or delay is made, use G-CSF 5 μg/kg SC for 5 days on odd weeks (after myelosuppressive drugs, so give on days 3–8 and 18–23).
- Prophylaxis: Bactrim double-strength bid, acyclovir 200 mg po tid, ketoconazole 200 mg daily, H-2 blocker daily, stool softener daily (equivalent drugs/doses acceptable).
- Two cycles (8 weeks) may be used for early stage disease.

■ References

Bartlett NL, Rosenberg SA, Hoppe RT, et al. Brief chemotherapy, Stanford V, and adjuvant radiotherapy for bulky or advanced-stage Hodgkin's disease: a preliminary report. *J Clin Oncol.* 1995;13(5):1080–1088.

Horning SJ, Williams J, Bartlett NL, et al. Assessment of the stanford V regimen and consolidative radiotherapy for bulky and advanced Hodgkin's disease: Eastern Cooperative Oncology Group pilot study E1492. *J Clin Oncol.* 2000;18(5):972–980.

BEACOPP *(and escalated BEACOPP): Every 3 weeks for eight cycles, followed by 30 Gy radiation to initial sites greater than 5 cm and 40 Gy to residual tumor sites.*

Agent	Dose	Days
Doxorubicin	25 (35) mg/m^2 IVP	1
Cyclophosphamide	650 (1,250) mg/m^2 IVPB	1
Etoposide	100 (200) mg/m^2 IVPB	1–3
Bleomycin	10 U/m^2 IVP	8
Vincristine	1.4 mg/m^2 (2 mg cap) IVP	8
Procarbazine	100 mg PO	1–7
Prednisone	40 mg/m^2 PO	1–14

■ Notes

* Etoposide may be given orally at double the IV dose.
* Prophylaxis with Bactrim, acyclovir.
* Escalated BEACOPP incorporates G-CSF support (starting at day 8, until WBC is normal), as does BEACOPP-14, a dose-dense version of regular BEACOPP (G-CSF on days 8–13).

■ References

Diehl V, Franklin J, Pfreundschuh M, et al. Standard and increased-dose BEACOPP chemotherapy compared with COPP-ABVD for advanced Hodgkin's disease. *N Engl J Med.* 2003;348(24):2386–2395.

Sieber M, Bredenfeld H, Josting A, et al. 14-day variant of the bleomycin, etoposide, doxorubicin, cyclophosphamide, vincristine, procarbazine, and prednisone regimen in advanced-stage Hodgkin's lymphoma: results of a pilot study of the German Hodgkin's Lymphoma Study Group. *J Clin Oncol.* 2003;21(9):1734–1739.

ChlVPP: *Every 4 weeks.*

Agent	Dose	Days
Vinblastine	6 mg/m^2 IV	1 and 8
Chlorambucil	6 mg/m^2 PO	1–14
Procarbazine	100 mg/m^2 PO	1–14
Prednisone	40 mg PO	1–14

■ Note

* ChlVPP is a pre-ABVD front-line chemotherapy regimen that is less intense and is less toxic than MOPP; often used in alternation with other regimens such as EVA (see below) or PABlOE; not standard.

■ References

Dady PJ, McElwain TJ, Austin DE, et al. Five years' experience with ChlVPP: effective low-toxicity combination chemotherapy for Hodgkin's disease. *Br J Cancer.* 1982;45(6): 851–859.

ChlVPP therapy for Hodgkin's disease: experience of 960 patients. The International ChlVPP Treatment Group. *Ann Oncol.* 1995;6(2):167–172.

Relapsed, Transplant Candidate: See "Relapsed Lymphoma" Section

Relapsed, Not a Transplant Candidate

Also see gemcitabine in "Relapsed Lymphoma" section.

EVA: *Every 4 weeks.*

Agent	Dose	Days
Etoposide	100 mg/m^2 IV	1–3
Vinblastine	6 mg/m^2 IV	1
Doxorubicin	50 mg/m^2 IV	1

■ Reference

Canellos GP, Petroni GR, Barcos M, et al. Etoposide, vinblastine, and doxorubicin: an active regimen for the treatment of Hodgkin's disease in relapse following MOPP. Cancer and Leukemia Group B. *J Clin Oncol.* 1995;13(8):2005–2011.

MINE: *Every 4 weeks.*

Agent	Dose	Days
Mitoguazone	500 mg/m^2	1 and 5
Ifosfamide	1500 mg/m^2	1–5
Vinorelbine	15 mg/m^2	1 and 5
Etoposide	150 mg/m^2	1–3

■ Reference

Ferme C, Bastion Y, Lepage E, et al. The MINE regimen as intensive salvage chemotherapy for relapsed and refractory Hodgkin's disease. *Ann Oncol.* 1995;6(6):543–549.

■ Non-Hodgkin's Lymphoma, Initial Treatment

Aggressive Lymphoma

(R-)CHOP-21: *Every 3 weeks.*

Agent	Dose	Days
Rituximab	375 mg/m^2 IV (over 3-5 hours)	1
Cyclophosphamide	750 mg/m^2 IVPB	1
Doxorubicin	50 mg/m^2 IVP	1
Vincristine	1.4 mg/m^2 (2 mg cap) IVP	1
Prednisone	100 mg PO	1–5

■ Notes

- Rituximab should be used only for B-cell malignancies.
- Prednisone dose variations include 40 mg/m^2, 60 mg/m^2, and 100 mg/m^2 days 1–5.
- G-CSF support should be considered for patients older than 60 years.
- "CNOP"—mitoxantrone 10 mg/m^2 substituted for doxorubicin.
- "CHEP"—etoposide 80 mg/m^2 days 1–3 substituted for vincristine.
- "CHOEP"—etoposide 100 mg/m^2 days 1–3 added to CHOP.

■ References

Fisher RI, Gaynor ER, Dahlberg S, et al. Comparison of a standard regimen (CHOP) with three intensive chemotherapy regimens for advanced non-Hodgkin's lymphoma. *N Engl J Med.* 1993; 328(14):1002–1006.

Coiffier B, Lepage E, Briere J, et al. CHOP chemotherapy plus rituximab compared with CHOP alone in elderly patients with diffuse large-B-cell lymphoma. *N Engl J Med.* 2002;346(4): 235–242.

(R-)CHOP-14 (accelerated)

Agent	Dose	Days
Rituximab	375 mg/m^2 IV (over 3–5 hours)	1
Cyclophosphamide	750 mg/m^2 IVPB	1
Doxorubicin	50 mg/m^2 IVP	1
Vincristine	1.4 mg/m^2 IVP (2-mg cap)	1
Prednisone	100 mg PO	1–5
G-CSF	5 mcg/kg	4–13

■ Notes

▪ Variations: Some centers use 1,000 mg/m^2 of cyclophosphamide instead of 750 mg/m^2; vincristine can be given as 2-mg flat dose; G-CSF duration varies.

▪ PCP prophylaxis with Bactrim.

■ Reference

Pfreundschuh M, Trumper L, Kloess M, et al. Two-weekly or 3-weekly CHOP chemotherapy with or without etoposide for the treatment of elderly patients with aggressive lymphomas: results of the NHL-B2 trial of the DSHNHL. *Blood.* 2004; 104(3):634–641.

ProMACE-CytaBOM: Every 3–4 weeks.

Agent	Dose	Days
ProMACE Prednisone	60 mg/m^2 PO	1–14
Doxorubicin	25 mg/m^2 IVP	1
Cyclophosphamide	650 mg/m^2 IVPB	1
Etoposide	120 mg/m^2 IVPB	1

Agent	Dose	Days
CytaBOM Cytarabine	300 mg/m^2 IVPB	8
Bleomycin	5 U/m^2 IVP	8
Vincristine	1.4 mg/m^2 IVP (2-mg cap)	8
Methotrexate (MTX)	120 mg/m^2 IVPB	8
Leucovorin	25 mg/m^2 PO	q6hr for 5 doses, start 24 hours after MTX

■ Notes

- ProMACE may be given alone on days 1 and 8.
- PCP prophylaxis.

■ Reference

Miller TP, Dahlberg S, Weick JK, et al. Unfavorable histologies of non-Hodgkin's lymphoma treated with ProMACE-CytaBOM: a groupwide Southwest Oncology Group study. *J Clin Oncol.* 1990;8(12):1951–1958.

(R-)CEPP(B): Every 4 weeks.

Agent	Dose	Days
Cyclophosphamide	600 mg/m^2 IVB	1
Etoposide	70 mg/m^2 IVPB	1
Etoposide	140 mg/m^2 PO	2–3
Procarbazine	60 mg/m^2 PO	1–10
Prednisone	60mg/m^2 PO	1–10
Cyclophosphamide	600 mg/m^2 IVB	8

■ Notes

* Anthracycline is not used, unlike most aggressive lymphoma regimens.
* Bleomycin (B) 15 U/m^2 IV on days 1 and 15 is usually omitted.

■ Reference

Chao NJ, Rosenberg SA, Horning SJ. CEPP(B): an effective and well-tolerated regimen in poor-risk, aggressive non-Hodgkin's lymphoma. *Blood.* 1990;76(7):1293–1298.

(R-)EPOCH: *Every 3 weeks.*

Agent	Dose	Days
Rituximab	375 mg/m² IV (over 3-5 hours)	1
Etoposide	50 mg/m²/day IVCI	1–4
Doxorubicin	10 mg/m²/day IVCI	1–4
Vincristine	0.4 mg/m²/day IVCI	1–4
Prednisone	60 mg/m² PO BID	1–5
Cyclophosphamide	750 mg/m² IVPB	6

■ Notes

* This infusional regimen usually is used in relapsed/refractory aggressive lymphoma, not to be confused with a bolus regimen CHOPE or CHOEP, which is usually used for untreated aggressive lymphoma.
* PCP prophylaxis with Bactrim.
* Dose adjustment performed based on absolute neutrophil count (ANC) but formalized subsequently in dose-adjusted EPOCH (DA-EPOCH), which is used in both newly diagnosed and relapsed/refractory aggressive lymphoma, usually with rituximab.

- DA-EPOCH increases doses of etoposide, doxorubicin, and cyclophosphamide by 20% to achieve nadir ANC of less than 500 for 1–2 measurements performed twice weekly at least 3 days apart in the previous cycle; GCSF 5μg/kg SC from day 6 until ANC is greater than 500.
- As stated before, (R-)DA-EPOCH can also be used in relapsed setting, usually without subsequent auto-transplantation.

■ References

Wilson WH, Bryant G, Bates S, et al. EPOCH chemotherapy: toxicity and efficacy in relapsed and refractory non-Hodgkin's lymphoma. *J Clin Oncol.* 1993;11(8):1573–1582.

Wilson WH, Grossbard ML, Pittaluga S, et al. Dose-adjusted EPOCH chemotherapy for untreated large B-cell lymphomas: a pharmacodynamic approach with high efficacy. *Blood.* 2002; 99(8):2685–2693.

Wilson WH, Gutierrez M, O'Connor P, et al. The role of rituximab and chemotherapy in aggressive B-cell lymphoma: a preliminary report of dose-adjusted EPOCH-R. *Seminars in Oncology.* 2002;29(1 Suppl 2):41–47.

Indolent Lymphoma
Single-Agent **Rituximab**

Agent	Dose	Days
Rituximab	375 mg/m^2 IV (over 3–5 hours)	1, 8, 15, and 22

■ Note

- Patients with high-circulating tumor cells (ALC greater than 20,000) are at greatest risk for infusion-related reactions. May split the dose by administering 100 mg IV on day 1 and the remainder of the calculated dose (375 mg/m^2 minus– 100 mg) on day 2.

■ References

Byrd JC, Waselenko JK, Maneatis TJ, et al. Rituximab therapy in hematologic malignancy patients with circulating blood tumor cells: association with increased infusion-related side effects and rapid blood tumor clearance. *J Clin Oncol.* 1999;17(3): 791–795.

McLaughlin P, Grillo-Lopez AJ, Link BK, et al. Rituximab chimeric anti-CD20 monoclonal antibody therapy for relapsed indolent lymphoma: half of patients respond to a four-dose treatment program. *J Clin Oncol.* 1998;16(8):2825–2833.

Rituximab with Chemotherapy on Day 1

- If ALC is less than 20,000 *and* if tolerated prior combination of rituximab and steroid-containing chemotherapy (e.g., CHOP, CVP) well, may infuse over 1.5 hours (Sehn LH, et al.) *or* if tolerated at least 2 prior rituximab doses within 3 months may infuse over 1 hour (Ghielmini M, et al.)
- With ALC greater than 20,000 or high tumor burden (e.g., bulky disease greater than 10 cm), split doses as per above and consider omitting rituximab from the first cycle.
- Often rituximab is given 1–2 days before chemotherapy because it is hard to fit all of the agents in a 1-day infusion.

Rituximab Maintenance Schedules

- Hainsworth et al.: Four weekly doses repeated every 6 months for 2 years (16 doses).
- Ghielmini et al.: One dose every 2 months for 8 months (4 doses).
- Van Oers et al.: One dose every 3 months for 2 years (8 doses).

■ Note

- Post-auto-transplant maintenance (Horwitz): Four weekly doses 6 weeks and 6 months after transplant (8 doses).

■ References

Ghielmini M, Negretti L, Lerch E, et al. Infusion speed-escalation trial to give full-dose rituximab in one hour without steroids pre-medication. *Blood*. 2005;106(11):2451a.

Ghielmini M, Negretti L, Lerch E, et al. Infusion speed-escalation trial to give full-dose rituximab in one hour without steroids pre-medication. *Blood*. 2005;106(11):2451a.

Ghielmini M, Schmitz SF, Cogliatti SB, et al. Prolonged treatment with rituximab in patients with follicular lymphoma significantly increases event-free survival and response duration compared with the standard weekly x 4 schedule. *Blood*. 2004; 103(12):4416–4423.

Hainsworth JD, Burris HA, 3rd, Morrissey LH, et al. Rituximab monoclonal antibody as initial systemic therapy for patients with low-grade non-Hodgkin lymphoma. *Blood*. 2000;95(10): 3052–3056.

Horwitz SM, Negrin RS, Blume KG, et al. Rituximab as adjuvant to high-dose therapy and autologous hematopoietic cell transplantation for aggressive non-Hodgkin lymphoma. *Blood*. 2004;103(3):777–783.

Sehn LH, Donaldson J, Filewich A, et al. Rapid infusion rituximab in combination with steroid containing chemotherapy can be given safely and substantially reduces resource utilization. *Blood*. 2004;104(11):1407a.

van Oers MH, Klasa R, Marcus RE, et al. Rituximab maintenance improves clinical outcome of relapsed/resistant follicular non-Hodgkin lymphoma in patients both with and without rituximab during induction: results of a prospective randomized phase 3 intergroup trial. *Blood*. 2006;108(10):3295–3301.

(R-)CVP: Every 3–4 weeks.

Agent	Dose	Days
Rituximab	375 mg/m^2 IV (over 3–5 hours)	1
Cyclophosphamide	750 mg/m^2 IVPB	1
Vincristine	1.4 mg/m^2 IVP (2 mg cap)	1
Prednisone	40 mg/m^2 PO	1–5

■ Notes

- What most people now call CVP is actually *COP*; original CVP used oral cyclophosphamide: 400 mg/m² PO days 1–5.
- Cyclophosphamide may be given at 1,000 mg/m².
- Prednisone may be given at 100 mg/m² on days 2–6 (as it was in COP) or at 100-mg flat dose.

■ Reference

Marcus R, Imrie K, Belch A, et al. CVP chemotherapy plus rituximab compared with CVP as first-line treatment for advanced follicular lymphoma. *Blood.* 2005;105(4):1417–1423.

Chlorambucil: Every 4 weeks.

Agent	Dose	Days
Chlorambucil	16 mg/m² PO	1–5

■ Notes

- Most commonly used for small lymphocytic lymphoma (SLL/CLL).
- There are many variations: chlorambucil may be given 4–8 mg/m² daily for 4–8 weeks or 15–40 mg/m² every 2–4 weeks, alone or with prednisone.

■ References

Cadman E, Drislane F, Waldron JA, Jr., et al. High-dose pulse chlorambucil: effective therapy for rapid remission induction in nodular lymphocytic poorly differentiated lymphoma. *Cancer.* 1982;50(6):1037–1041.

Rai KR, Peterson BL, Appelbaum FR, et al. Fludarabine compared with chlorambucil as primary therapy for chronic lymphocytic leukemia. *N Engl J Med.* 2000;343(24):1750–1757.

Cladribine: Every 4 weeks.

Agent	Dose	Days
Cladribine (2-CDA)	0.12 mg/kg IVPB over 2 hours	1–5

■ Notes

■ Longer treatment is the traditional regimen : 0.1 mg/kg/day IVCI days 1–7.
■ Drug of choice for hairy-cell leukemia, where one cycle may induce a durable remission.

■ References

Piro LD, Carrera CJ, Carson DA, Beutler E. Lasting remissions in hairy-cell leukemia induced by a single infusion of 2-chlorodeoxyadenosine. *N Engl J Med.* 1990;322(16):1117–1121.

Robak T, Blonski JZ, Kasznicki M, et al. Cladribine with or without prednisone in the treatment of previously treated and un-treated B-cell chronic lymphocytic leukaemia - updated results of the multicentre study of 378 patients. *Br J Haematol.* 2000;108(2):357–368.

(R-)FC: *Every 4 weeks.*

Agent	Dose	Days
Rituximab	375 mg/m^2 IV (over 3-5 hours)	1
Fludarabine	20 mg/m^2 IVPB	1–5
Cyclophosphamide	1,000 mg/m^2 IVPB	1

■ Notes

■ Cyclophosphamide may be given at 600 mg/m^2.
■ G-CSF starts day 8 for 10–14 days.
■ All fludarabine-containing regimens should receive PCP prophylaxis; herpes zoster prophylaxis should be considered.
■ May give allopurinol with the first cycle for tumor lysis prophylaxis.

■ References

Flinn IW, Byrd JC, Morrison C, et al. Fludarabine and cyclophosphamide with filgrastim support in patients with previously untreated indolent lymphoid malignancies. *Blood.* 2000;96(1):71–75.

Hochster HS, Oken MM, Winter JN, et al. Phase I study of flu-darabine plus cyclophosphamide in patients with previously untreated low-grade lymphoma: results and and long-term fol-low-up—a report from the Eastern Cooperative Oncology Group. *J Clin Oncol.* 2000;18(5):987–994.

(R-)FND: *Every 4 weeks.*

Agent	Dose	Days
Rituximab	375 mg/m^2 IV (over 3–5 hours)	1
Fludarabine	25 mg/m^2 IVPB	1–3
Mitoxantrone (Novantrone)	10 mg/m^2 IV	1
Dexamethasone	20 mg PO	1–4

■ Note

* "FN"—no dexamethasone.
* Fludarabine alone can be given with or without rituximab at 25mg/m^2 days 1–5 (longer duration).
* PCP prophylaxis.

■ References

McLaughlin P, Hagemeister FB, Rodriguez MA, et al. Safety of fludarabine, mitoxantrone, and dexamethasone combined with rituximab in the treatment of stage IV indolent lymphoma. *Seminars in Oncology.* 2000;27(6 Suppl 12):37–41.

McLaughlin P, Hagemeister FB, Swan F, Jr., et al. Phase I study of the combination of fludarabine, mitoxantrone, and dexam-ethasone in low-grade lymphoma. *J Clin Oncol.* 1994;12(3):575–579.

(R-)FCM: *Every 4 weeks.*

Agent	Dose	Days
Rituximab	375 mg/m^2 IV (over 3-5 hours)	1
Fludarabine	25 mg/m^2 IVPB	2–4
Cyclophosphamide	200 mg/m^2 IVPB	2–4
Mitoxantrone	8 mg/m^2 IV	2

■ Notes

■ Variations include mitoxantrone 10 mg/m^2 (as in FND) and cyclophosphamide 300 mg/m^2.
■ Can be used in relapsed mantle cell lymphoma.

■ Reference

Forstpointner R, Dreyling M, Repp R, et al. The addition of rituximab to a combination of fludarabine, cyclophosphamide, mitoxantrone (FCM) significantly increases the response rate and prolongs survival as compared with FCM alone in patients with relapsed and refractory follicular and mantle cell lymphomas: results of a prospective randomized study of the German Low-Grade Lymphoma Study Group. *Blood.* 2004;104(10): 3064–3071.

Initial Treatment, Highly Aggressive Lymphoma (Burkitt's)

CODOX-M/IVAC (Magrath): *Alternate regimens A/B/A/B every 3–4 weeks.*

Regimen A: CODOX-M

Agent	Dose	Days
Cyclophosphamide	800 mg/m^2 IVPB 200 mg/m^2 IVPB	1 days 2–5
Vincristine	1.5 mg/m^2 IVP	days 1 and 8*
Doxorubicin	40 mg/m^2 IVP	1

Agent	Dose	Days
Methotrexate (MTX)	1,200 mg/m^2 IVPB (over 1 hour) then 240 mg/m^2/hr IVCI over 23 hours	10
Leucovorin	192 mg/m^2 IVPB and then 12 mg/m^2 IVPB/PO q6h until MTX level is less than 5×10^{-8}mol/L	36 hours after MTX started
IT Cytarabine	70 mg IT	1 and 3
IT Methotrexate	12 mg IT	15

■ Notes

- ▪ *Give additional dose of vincristine in cycle 3, day 15.
- ▪ G-CSF 5 mcg/kg SC daily starting day 13 until ANC is greater than 1,000.
- ▪ Three doses of modified CODOX-M are given to low-risk patients with normal LDH and single extra-abdominal mass or resected abdominal disease. There is no day 15 vincristine or G-CSF; IT Cytarabine is given on day 1 and IT MTX on day 3.

Regimen B: IVAC

Agent	Dose	Days
Ifosfamide	1,500 mg/m^2 IV	1–5
Mesna	360 mg/m^2 IVPB q3h	1–5
Etoposide	60 mg/m^2 IVPB	1–5
Cytarabine	2000 mg/m^2 IVPB q12h x 4	1–2
IT Methotrexate	12 mg IT	5

■ Notes

- ▣ G-CSF 5 mcg/kg SC daily starting day 7 until ANC is greater than 1,000.
- ▣ Steroid eye drops with cytarabine.

■ Reference

Magrath I, Adde M, Shad A, et al. Adults and children with small non-cleaved-cell lymphoma have a similar excellent outcome when treated with the same chemotherapy regimen. *J Clin Oncol.* 1996;14(3):925–934.

Initial Treatment, Mantle Cell Lymphoma and Burkitt's
(R-)Hyper-CVAD/(R-)M-A: *Alternate regimens A/B/A/B/A/B/A/B every 3 weeks.*

Regimen A: (R-)HyperCVAD

Agent	Dose	Days
Rituximab	375 mg/m² IV (over 3–5 hours)	1
Cyclophosphamide	300 mg/m² IV q12h × 6	2–4
Doxorubicin	25 mg/m² IVCI	5–6
Vincristine	2 mg IV	5*,12
Dexamethasone	40 mg IV/PO	2–5,12–15

■ Notes

- ▣ *Start 12 hours after last cyclophosphamide dose.
- ▣ G-CSF 5 mcg/kg IV/SC daily starting 24 hours after the end of doxorubicin infusion until WBC is greater than 4500.

Regimen B: (R-)M-A

Agent	Dose	Days
Rituximab	375 mg/m^2 IV (over 3–5 hours)	1
Methotrexate (MTX)	200 mg/m^2 IVP Then 800 mg/m^2 IVCI over 24 hours	2
Folinic acid	50 mg PO then 15 mg* PO q6h × 8	24 hours after end of MTX
Cytarabine	3,000 mg/m^2 IV q12h × 4	3-4

■ Notes

- *Folinic acid dose adjusted to MTX level taken at 24 and 48 hours after MTX completion.
- Decrease cytarabine to 1,000 mg/m^2 in patients older than 60 years or Cr greater than 1.5 mg/dL.
- G-CSF 5 mcg/kg IV/SC daily starting 24 hours after chemotherapy completion until WBC greater than 4,500.
- Steroid eye drops starting with cytarabine for 7 days.
- Staging every two cycles (four treatments).
- Prophylaxis with valacyclovir, fluconazole, and levofloxacin/ciprofloxacin.
- For Burkitt's, hyper-CVAD/M-A includes IT prophylaxis with MTX 12 mg day 2 and cytarabine 100 mg day 7 of each regimen; rituximab was given on days 1 and 11 of hyper-CVAD and days 2 and 8 of M-A only during the first four regimens.

■ References

MCL

Khouri IF, Romaguera J, Kantarjian H, et al. Hyper-CVAD and high-dose methotrexate/cytarabine followed by stem-cell transplantation: an active regimen for aggressive mantle-cell lymphoma. *J Clin Oncol.* 1998;16(12):3803–3809.

Romaguera JE, Fayad L, Rodriguez MA, et al. High rate of durable remissions after treatment of newly diagnosed aggressive mantle-cell lymphoma with rituximab plus hyper-CVAD alternating with rituximab plus high-dose methotrexate and cytarabine. *J Clin Oncol.* 2005;23(28):7013–7023.

Burkitt's

Thomas DA, Cortes J, O'Brien S, et al. Hyper-CVAD program in Burkitt's-type adult acute lymphoblastic leukemia. *J Clin Oncol.* 1999;17(8):2461–2470.

Thomas DA, Faderl S, O'Brien S, et al. Chemoimmunotherapy with hyper-CVAD plus rituximab for the treatment of adult Burkitt and Burkitt-type lymphoma or acute lymphoblastic leukemia. *Cancer.* 2006;106(7):1569–1580.

Relapsed/Refractory Lymphoma

(R-)ICE: Every 2 weeks for two (HL) or three (NHL) cycles.

Agent	Dose	Days
Rituximab	375 mg/m² IV (over 3–5 hours)	1
Etoposide	100 mg/m² IVPB	1–3
Ifosfamide (IFOS)	5,000 mg/m² IVCI over 24 hours	2
Mesna (mixed with IFOS)	5,000 mg/m² IVCI over 24 hours	2
Carboplatin	AUC 5 IVPB (800-mg cap)	2

■ Notes

- *Rituximab also given day 2 in cycle 1.
- Carboplatin dosing based on Calvert formula (AUC × creatinine clearance + 25) from 12-hour creatinine clearance initiated day 1.
- Cycle 1 (and 2 for NHL) delayed if ANC less than 1,000 and platelets less than 50K.

- Intended to be given q14 days; average is q17 days with delays.
- G-CSF 5 mcg/kg SC daily on days 5–12 in cycle 1 (and 2 for NHL).
- G-CSF 10 mcg/kg SC daily from day 5 until stem cell collection complete (last cycle).
- Regimen followed by autotransplant.
- Augmented ICE: doubles the doses of ifosfamide, mesna, and etoposide. Ifosfamide and mesna 5,000 mg/m^2 both days 1 and 2; etoposide 200 mg/m^2 q12h × 3 doses days 1 and 2.
- Prophylaxis with acyclovir, fluconazole, Bactrim, ciprofloxacin.

■ References

Moskowitz CH, Bertino JR, Glassman JR, et al. Ifosfamide, carboplatin, and etoposide: a highly effective cytoreduction and peripheral-blood progenitor-cell mobilization regimen for transplant-eligible patients with non-Hodgkin's lymphoma. *J Clin Oncol.* 1999;17(12):3776–3785.

Moskowitz CH, Nimer SD, Zelenetz AD, et al. A 2-step comprehensive high-dose chemoradiotherapy second-line program for relapsed and refractory Hodgkin disease: analysis by intent to treat and development of a prognostic model. *Blood.* 2001; 97(3):616–623.

(R-)DHAP: *Every 3–4 weeks for two to six cycles.*

Agent	Dose	Days
Rituximab	375 mg/m^2 IV (over 3-5 hours)	1
Cisplatin	100 mg/m^2 IVCI	1
Cytarabine	2,000 mg/m^2 IVPB q12h × 2	2
Dexamethasone	40 mg IV/PO	1–4

◼ Notes

▪ Steroid eye drops starting with cytarabine until 2–3 days after its completion.
▪ Regimen followed by autotransplant.

◼ Reference

Velasquez WS, Cabanillas F, Salvador P, et al. Effective salvage therapy for lymphoma with cisplatin in combination with high-dose Ara-C and dexamethasone (DHAP). *Blood.* 1988;71(1): 117–122.

ESHAP : *Every 3 weeks.*

Agent	Dose	Days
Etoposide	40 mg/m² IV (over 1 hour)	1–4
Methylprednisolone	500 mg/m² IV (over 15 min)	1–5
Cisplatin	25 mg/m²/day IVCI	1–4
Cytarabine	2,000 mg/m² IV (over 2 hours)	5

◼ Notes

▪ Administer cytarabine after completing cisplatin infusion.
▪ In a variant that was published subsequently, etoposide dose was increased to 60 mg/m² and Solumedrol was given only for 4 days.
▪ ESHAP is most commonly used in NHL without subsequent autotransplant, but there are publications for HL and for autotransplant settings.
▪ "ASHAP" replaced etoposide with doxorubicin 10 mg/m²/d IVCI days 1–4.

◼ Reference

Velasquez WS, McLaughlin P, Tucker S, et al. ESHAP—an effective chemotherapy regimen in refractory and relapsing lymphoma: a 4-year follow-up study. *J Clin Oncol.* 1994;12(6):1169–1176.

Dexa-BEAM: Every 4 weeks for 2-5 cycles.

Agent	Dose	Days
Dexamethasone	8 mg PO q8h	1–10
BCNU	60 mg/m^2 IVPB	2
Melphalan	20 mg/m^2 IVPB	3
Etoposide	150 mg/m^2 IVPB	4–7
Cytarabine	100 mg/m^2 IVPB	4–7

■ Notes

- Etoposide dose varies from 75 to 250 mg/m^2.
- G-CSF given from day 8 until leukocyte recovery or sufficient stem cell collection.
- Regimen followed by autotransplant; mostly used in HL, but also in mantle cell and indolent lymphomas.
- "Mini-BEAM" omits dexamethasone; "BEAM" is a standard high-dose chemotherapy prior to autotransplant.

■ References

Josting A, Reiser M, Wickramanayake PD, et al. Dexamethasone, carmustine, etoposide, cytarabine, and melphalan (dexa-BEAM) followed by high-dose chemotherapy and stem cell rescue—a highly effective regimen for patients with refractory or relapsed indolent lymphoma. *Leukemia & Lymphoma.* 2000; 37(1–2):115–123.

Pfreundschuh MG, Rueffer U, Lathan B, et al. Dexa-BEAM in patients with Hodgkin's disease refractory to multidrug chemotherapy regimens: a trial of the German Hodgkin's Disease Study Group. *J Clin Oncol.* 1994;12(3):580–586.

Gemcitabine: Every 4 weeks.

Agent	Dose	Days
Gemcitabine	1,250 mg/m^2 IV	days 1,8,15

■ Notes

▪ Can also be given at 1,000 mg/m^2, particularly if given in combinations with other drugs. "GDP"—gemcitabine 1,000 mg/m^2 IV days 1 and 8, cisplatin 75 mg/m^2 IV day 1, and dexamethasone 40 mg PO days 1–4, given every 3 weeks.

▪ "GVD"—gemcitabine 1,000 mg/m^2 IV days 1 and 8, vinorelbine 20 mg/m^2 IV days 1 and 8, and liposomal doxorubicin 10 mg/m^2 IV days 1 and 8, given every 3 weeks.

▪ Mostly used in HL, may be given in relapse after autotransplant; palliative as a single agent, but GDP and GVD may be used prior to autotransplant.

■ References

Fossa A, Santoro A, Hiddemann W, et al. Gemcitabine as a single agent in the treatment of relapsed or refractory aggressive non-Hodgkin's lymphoma. *J Clin Oncol.* 1999;17(12):3786–3792.

Santoro A, Bredenfeld H, Devizzi L, et al. Gemcitabine in the treatment of refractory Hodgkin's disease: results of a multicenter phase II study. *J Clin Oncol.* 2000;18(13):2615–2619.

Bortezomib: *Every 3 weeks.*

Agent	Dose	Days
Bortezomib	1.3 mg/m^2	1, 4, 8, 11

■ Note

▪ Used in relapsed mantle cell lymphoma and sometimes follicular lymphoma.

■ Reference

Fisher RI, Bernstein SH, Kahl BS, et al. Multicenter phase II study of bortezomib in patients with relapsed or refractory mantle cell lymphoma. *J Clin Oncol.* 2006;24(30):4867–4874.

CHAPTER 8

Cutaneous T-cell Lymphoma: Mycosis Fungoides and Sézary Syndrome

■ Epidemiology

- A diverse category of rare lymphomas with a different treatment paradigm
- Primary cutaneous lymphomas involve skin only as initial site of disease.
- New consensus classification of cutaneous lymphomas was published in 2005[1] (table 8-1).
- Primary cutaneous lymphomas have a different behavior from histologically similar nodal lymphoma.
  - Primary cutaneous anaplastic large cell lymphoma and what often appears to be diffuse large B-cell lymphoma (non-leg-type) and is now called primary cutaneous follicle center lymphoma have histologically aggressive appearance but an indolent course.
  - Similarly, lymphomatoid papulomatosis may appear histologically aggressive (especially type C) but has an indolent course.
  - The key is not to overtreat based on histology alone but to look at clinical behavior for guidance.
- Estimated incidence of primary skin involvement by lymphoma is 1:100,000.
- Cutaneous T-cell lymphomas (CTCLs) represent about 80% of all cutaneous lymphomas, while cutaneous B-cell lymphomas represent about 20%.
- Most common CTCL is mycosis fungoides (MF).
  - MF and its variants represented about 50% of all primary cutaneous lymphomas and 65% of CTCL in a series of 1905 patients.[1]
  - The next most common subtype is lymphomatoid papulosis (12%).

Table 8-1: Relative Frequency and Disease-specific 5-Year Survival of 1905 Primary Cutaneous Lymphomas Classified According to the WHO-EORTC Classification

WHO-EORTC classification	No.	Frequency, %*	Disease-specific 5-year survival, %
Cutaneous T-cell lymphoma			
Indolent clinical behavior			
Mycosis fungoides	800	44	88
Folliculotropic MF	86	4	80
Pagetoid reticulosis	14	<1	100
Granulomatous slack skin	4	<1	100
Primary cutaneous anaplastic large cell lymphoma	146	8	95
Lymphomatoid papulosis	236	12	100
Subcutaneous panniculitis-like T-cell lymphoma	18	1	82
Primary cutaneous CD4+ small/medium pleomorphic T-cell lymphoma[†]	39	2	75
Aggressive clinical behavior			
Sézary syndrome	52	3	24
Primary cutaneous NK/T-cell lymphoma, nasal-type	7	<1	NR
Primary cutaneous aggressive CD8+ T-cell lymphoma[†]	14	<1	18
Primary cutaneous γ/δ T-cell lymphoma[†]	13	<1	NR
Primary cutaneous peripheral T-cell lymphoma, unspecified[‡]	47	2	16

Cutaneous B-cell lymphoma

Indolent clinical behavior			
Primary cutaneous marginal zone B-cell lymphoma	127	7	99
Primary cutaneous follicle center lymphoma	207	11	95
Intermediate clinical behavior			
Primary cutaneous diffuse large B-cell lymphoma, leg type	85	4	55
Primary cutaneous diffuse large B-cell lymphoma, other	4	< 1	50
Primary cutaneous intravascular large B-cell lymphoma	6	< 1	65

NR Indicates not reached.

*Data are based on 1905 patients with a primary cutaneous lymphoma registered at The Dutch and Austrian Cutaneous Lymphoma Group between 1986 and 2002.

†Primary cutaneous peripheral T-cell lymphoma, unspecified excluding the three provisional entities indicated with a double dagger (‡).

Source: Willemze R, Jaffe ES, Burg G, et al: *Blood*; 2005;105(10):3768–3785.

- Sézary syndrome (SS) is a disease closely related to MF where malignant cells present in the skin also involve the blood at diagnosis.
  - about 5% of MF incidence
- This discussion will focus on MF.
- An indolent-behaving subtype with slow progression over a period of many years
- Death is usually from infections or systemic involvement.
- Incidence 3:1,000,000; 1500–2000 cases per year
- Median age is 55–60, with 2:1 male-to-female ratio, and increased incidence in African-Americans
- Etiology unclear, with possible contribution of chemicals and HTLV-1

■ Presentation

- Skin symptoms often predate diagnosis by several years, because appearance may be nonspecific and biopsies non-diagnostic.
- Initially presents in the "bathing suit" areas (trunk, buttocks, inguinal areas), in advanced stages becomes diffuse
- Progresses from erythematous scaly patches to plaques and then to tumors, and sometimes to erythroderma, which is also seen in SS.
  - Patches are flat while plaques are raised, thicker, and may be ulcerated.
  - Tumors are deeper, at least 1 cm in greatest diameter, and mostly involve the dermis.
  - Erythroderma is generalized (at least 80% of body surface area) reddening and scaling, often with severe itching.
- Large tumors look like fungus (mushroom), hence the name "mycosis fungoides."
- SS is a combination of erythroderma, lymphadenopathy, and Sézary (lymphoma) cells in peripheral blood. It has very poor prognosis.
  - The name Sézary syndrome should be reserved for patients that present with the above characteristics at diagnosis. If patients develop MF and then later progress to have the above characteristics, it should be termed erythrodermic MF.

■ Pathology

Morphology

- Epidermis (commonly its basal layer) is infiltrated by small- to medium-sized T-lymphocytes with "cerebriform" (convoluted, like the brain surface) nuclei.
- When such atypical lymphocytes form clusters in the epidermis, they are called Pautrier microabsesses.
  - They are pathognomonic for MF but are not necessary for the diagnosis.
  - They are more prominent in plaque rather than patch stage.
- Other features of atypical lymphocytes include perinuclear haloes and linear infiltration of the basal epidermal layer.
- With progression to tumor stage, this predilection for epidermis (epidermotropism) is lost, and the deeper dermal infiltration predominates.
  - The lymphocytes display greater numbers and variability in size, with occasional blasts.
- Histologic involvement of lymph nodes is graded according to the Dutch system[2] or the National Cancer Institute/Veterans Administration, with the latter shown below:[3,4]
  - Category I (LN0–2) has no or small clusters (up to 6 cells) of atypical lymphocytes with cerebriform nuclei.
  - Category II (LN3) shows focal infiltration with clusters of more than 6 cells.
  - Category III (LN4) shows complete effacement by such lymphocytes.
  - Only categories II and III count as lymph node involvement.
  - LN4 is prognostically worse than LN3.
- Transformation to large cell lymphoma
  - Usually occurs in tumor (T3) stage
  - Atypical large lymphocytes, at least 4 times the size of normal lymphocytes, present in at least 25% of the dermal infiltrate
  - May be CD30 positive or negative
  - Poor prognosis
  - Treatment varies but often combines localized and systemic therapies (see below).

■ Immunophenotype

- MF cells have memory T-cell phenotype: CD3+, CD4+, CD8−, CD45RO+
- Rarely they can be CD4−, CD8+ (cytotoxic rather than helper phenotype).
- Loss of pan T-cell antigens is frequent (CD2, CD3, CD5, or CD7).
- Neoplastic cells in more advanced disease may express cytotoxic proteins such as granzyme B and TIA-1.

■ Cytogenetic and Molecular Changes

- Most cases have clonal T-cell receptor (TCR) rearrangements.
- Chromosomal aberrations are found in majority of cases and increase with advanced stage.
- Chromosomal losses at 6q, 10q, and 13q, and gains at 7 and 8q; and inactivation of tumor suppressors p15, p16, and p53 can be detected.[5]
- Gene expression profile of MF demonstrated the importance of TNF anti-apoptotic pathway and found a 27-gene signature.[6]
- SS shows predominance of genes associated with Th2 T-cell response (elaborating IL-4, IL-5, IL-10), even with minimal blood involvement.[7]

■ Staging

- Staging is by tumor, node, metastasis model,[8] as in solid tumors, and was recently updated:[9]
  - T1 is limited patch/plaque, with <10% total skin area involvement, while T2 is diffuse patch/plaque with ≥10% total skin area involvement, T3 is tumors, and T4 is erythroderma.
  - N0 is no lymph node involvement, N1 is clinically but not histologically involved, N2 is histologically but not clinically involved (i.e., not enlarged), and N3 represents both clinically and histologically involved lymph nodes.
    - Recently updated definition acknowledges that clinically uninvolved lymph nodes are no longer routinely biopsied and proposes that N2 nodes should be defined as clinically abnormal lymph

nodes with LN3 histology and N3 as enlarged lymph nodes with LN4 histology.

- ▪ Pathologic size is determined as at least 1.5 cm in greatest diameter or any palpable lymph node.
- ● M1 denotes visceral histologic involvement (usually liver, spleen, lung, or bone marrow).
  - ▪ Note that in cutaneous lymphomas spleen is a metastatic organ, unlike in Ann Arbor staging for systemic lymphomas.
- ● Suffix B (not to be confused with stage B) is given for blood involvement by Sézary cells.
  - ▪ B0 is defined as less than 5% of lymphocytes being Sézary cells.
  - ▪ B1 is defined as at least 5% of lymphocytes being Sézary cells.
  - ▪ B2 meets definition of overt peripheral blood involvement, as in SS.
  - ▪ New guidelines propose using the suffix for staging purposes.
- ▪ The more extensive the cutaneous involvement, the greater the probability of extracutaneous spread.
  - ● In a series of 434 patients with skin-only disease, the 20-year probability of extracutaneous progression was 0% for T1, 10% for T2, 36% for T3, and 41% for T4 disease.[10]
- ▪ Stage IA (T1) patients have excellent survival that may not even be affected by disease.[10a]
- ▪ Stage IB (T2) and IIA (T1/2 and N1) patients have intermediate survival.[10a]
- ▪ Stage IIB (T3), III (T4), and IV (N2/N3, and/or M1) patients have poor long-term survival.[10a]
  - ● T3 patients may actually fare worse than T4 patients.
- ▪ Updated staging guidelines propose grouping N2 with N1 and using B2 to define stage IV disease.
- ▪ Criteria for diagnosis of peripheral blood involvement in SS, as per International Society for Cutaneous Lymphoma are:[11]
  - ● More than 1,000/mm^3 of atypical T lymphocytes with cerebriform nuclei (Sézary cells), or/and
  - ● By flow cytometry with highly skewed CD4/CD8 ratio of ≥10 and/or loss of pan-T cell markers (CD2, CD3, CD4, CD5), or/and

- By demonstration of clonality by molecular or cytogenetic means
- Recent update uses TCR gene rearrangement plus either of the first two criteria to define B2 peripheral blood involvement.

■ Workup

- Biopsy and dermatopathology review critical in diagnosis
  - Skin biopsy should include immunophenotyping and clonality assessment for TCR gene rearrangement.
  - Importance of clonality assessment on lymph node biopsies is uncertain.
- In all patients:
  - Full skin exam with determination of percentage of body surface area (BSA) involvement by patches/plaques and size measurements of tumors
    - Palm alone is about 0.5% BSA.
  - Assessment for lymphadenopathy and hepatosplenomegaly
- T1—Complete blood count with manual review for Sézary cells and a chest X-ray
- T2 and above—peripheral blood flow cytometry or TCR gene rearrangement to look for Sézary cells
  - Additional workup should include lactate dehydrogenase, comprehensive metabolic panel, computerized tomography (CT) chest/abdomen/pelvis +/− positron-emission tomography/CT, excisional biopsy of suspicious lymph nodes, biopsy of visceral lesions (except the spleen, which may be considered involved on clinical grounds).
  - Bone marrow biopsy is not required for staging.
  - Additional laboratories/investigations depending on type of treatment being considered (see below)

■ Prognosis

- Stage is the most important prognostic factor, with the groupings as noted above.
- Presence of lymph node, blood, and visceral involvement; complex cytogenetic abnormalities; and transformation to large cell lymphoma are unfavorable.

■ Treatment

* Therapies can be broken down into localized (skin-directed or topical) and systemic.
* Skin-directed treatments include:
  * Topical corticosteroids
  * Topical chemotherapy (mechlorethamine or carmustine)
  * Topical retinoids (bexarotene, tazarotene)
  * Phototherapy (PUVA or ultraviolet B [UVB])
  * Localized radiation (electron beam therapy, EBT)
  * Total skin electron beam therapy (TSEBT)
* Systemic therapies include:
  * Interferon (alpha and gamma)
  * Retinoids (bexarotene, 13-sis, acitretin, all-trans retinoid acid [ATRA])
  * Extracorporeal photophoresis (ECP)
  * Histone deacetylase (HDAC) inhibitor (vorinostat)
  * Denileukin diftitox
  * Single-agent chemotherapy (methotrexate, gemcitabine, liposomal doxorubicin, chlorambucil (+steroid), pentostatin, alemtuzumab)
  * Combination chemotherapy (cyclosphosharnide, doxorubicin, and prednisone [CHOP])
* A combination of localized and systemic therapies is often used.

■ Skin-directed Treatment

* Most studies of skin-directed treatments are limited by retrospective analysis and lack of placebo controls.
  * An exception was a randomized double-blind placebo-controlled trial of topical peldesine, a purine nucleoside phosphorylase inhibitor, in stage IA/IB patients.
  * Response was seen in 28% of patients receiving peldesine but also in 24% of patients receiving a placebo vehicle cream (p=0.677).[12]
  * The drug has not been approved for use.
* Additional difficulty is assessing response, relying on visual inspection and meticulous measurement of percent BSA involved.

- Most studies define complete remission (CR) as resolution of all lesions, partial remission (PR) as at least 50% reduction of lesion area, for at least 4 weeks.
  - Some studies use reduction in target lesions only, or in specific measurement scores.
- Progression is often defined as 25% increase in lesions, progression to a higher T stage, or new lymph node/visceral findings.
- Physician's Global Assessment and composite assessment are commonly used scales,[13] but other assessment schemes exist.
- Topical corticosteroids
  - Moderate-to-strong potency steroids used (classes III-I)
    - E.g., clobetazol 0.05%, triamcinolone 0.1%
  - One study of 79 patients showed 63% CR in T1 patients and 25% in T2 patients.[14]
  - Response duration may be short, particularly with more extensive disease.
  - Side effects: erythema, striae, atrophy
- Topical chemotherapy
  - Topical mechlorethamine (nitrogen mustard)
    - No systemic absorption
    - CR 65–80%, time to achieve CR several months (may be over a year in T2 disease), 20–25% durable response[15]
    - Maintenance of several months is often used, but the evidence for it is unclear.
    - Side effects: contact hypersensitivity (aqueous >ointment), irritation
      - Secondary skin cancer unusual in monotherapy
  - Topical carmustine (BCNU)
    - Efficacy similar to mechlorethamine
      - In a report of 15-year experience with 143 patients, carmustine produced CR in 86% of patients with T1 and in 47% of patients with T2 disease (and even 21% of patients with T4 disease).
      - Median time to CR was 11.5 weeks.[16]
    - Side effects: systemic absorption with bone marrow suppression, telangiectasias, erythema

- ▨ Risk of secondary skin cancer unclear
- ▨ Topical retinoids (bexarotene, tazarotene)
  - • Bexarotene (1% gel)
    - ▨ Phase I/II trial of 67 patients in stages IA-IIA showed 63% overall response rate (ORR), 21% CR, median time to response of 20.1 weeks, median response duration 99 weeks.[17]
  - • Tazarotene (0.1%): 58% ORR, 35% CR in a pilot trial of 19 patients[18]
  - • Side effects: skin irritation; expensive
- ▨ Phototherapy
  - • Psoralen + UVA photochemotherapy (PUVA)
    - ▨ Most commonly used phototherapy and one of the most frequently used localized treatments
    - ▨ Oral psoralen followed 2 hours later by UVA radiation
    - ▨ Psoralen intercalates with DNA and then cross-links it upon UVA exposure
    - ▨ Given 3 times a week until complete remission, often followed by maintenance taper
    - ▨ Two studies of 82 patients showed overall CR of 62–65%, with 79–88% CR in stage IA (T1) and 52–59% in stage IB (T2) disease.
      - • There were CRs in more advanced stages: 83% in stage IIA (T1–2N1) and 46% in stage III (T4).[19,20]
    - ▨ Long-term follow-up of 66 stage IA-IIA patients achieving CR reported that 50% of patients maintained median CR of 7 years, while the other 50% relapsed at a median disease-free interval of 3.3 years.
      - • DFS rates at 5 and 10 years with stage IA were 56% and 30%, respectively, and for stage IB/IIA, 74% and 50%, respectively.
      - • Overall survival (OS) rates at 5, 10, and 15 years with stage IA were 94%, 82%, and 82%, respectively, and for stage IB/IIA, 80%, 69%, and 58%, respectively.[21]
    - ▨ Side effects: xerosis, erythema, pruritus, nausea
      - • Increased risk of secondary skin cancers including melanoma[21]
      - • Cataracts
    - ▨ May be combined with interferon (IFN) or with retinoids (see below)

- UVB
  - Limited penetration, best for patches or thin plaques
  - Broadband UVB (290–310 nm) showed CR of 71%, with CRs limited to patch but not plaque disease, in a small series of 35 patients
    - Median time to response 5 months, duration of response 22 months[22]
  - Narrowband UVB (311–313 nm) was retrospectively compared to PUVA in 21 stage IA and IB patients.
    - 81% CR, 19% PR, duration of remission 24.5 months, as compared to 71% CR, 29% PR, duration of remission 22.8 months in 35 patients with PUVA[23]
    - Expected to be less carcinogenic
- Local radiation (EBT)
  - Appropriate for single lesions
  - An older retrospective study of 20 patients with 191 lesions reported 95% CR in patch stage and in tumors less than 3 cm in diameter, and 93% CR in tumors greater than 3 cm.
  - All patients receiving at least 20 Gy of radiation responded, and no patient receiving at least 30 Gy relapsed in the radiation field.[24]
  - Side effects: xerosis, erythema, telangiectasias
- TSEBT
  - Appropriate for more disseminated cutaneous disease, stages IB/IIA
  - Meta-analysis of 952 patients showed 96% CR in T1–2, 36% in T3, and 60% in T4 disease, with higher radiation doses and higher electron voltage resulting in higher CR rates.[25]
  - TSEBT vs. topical mechlorethamine: randomized controlled trial of 42 patients showed that in early stages the modalities are equally effective but in later stages (short of stage IV) TSEBT results in better overall response.[26]
    - Considering the side effect profile, topical mechlorethamine would be preferred in earlier stage disease and TSEBT can be used in later stages.

* Side effects: xerosis, erythema, telangiectasias, pruritus, anhidrosis, nail loss, secondary skin cancers

■ Systemic Treatment

* IFN (alpha and gamma)
  * IFN alpha (2a and 2b)—no difference in activity between the two
    * Administered 3 times a week, typically starting at 1–3 million units a day, titrated up for response and toxicity
    * ORR 30–75%, commonly around 50%, few CRs, with variable duration of response
    * IFN alpha with PUVA: 39 patients in a phase I/II trial with stage IB–IVB disease had CR of 62% and PR of 28% with median duration of response 28 months and median survival of 62 months.[27]
      * Maximum tolerated dose of IFN alpha was 12 million units 3 times a week.
  * IFN gamma: 16 patients with mostly advanced disease had 31% PR with median duration of 10 months.[28]
  * Side effects: flu-like symptoms, fatigue, depression, anorexia, cytopenias, elevated transaminases
* Retinoids (bexarotene, isotretinoin, acitretin, etretinate, ATRA)
  * Vitamin A derivatives signaling either through retinoid acid receptor in the case of older retinoids, or retinoid X receptor in the case of bexarotene
  * With older retinoids ORR ranged from 44 to 80% and CR from 12 to 30%.
  * Side effects: xerosis, cheilitis, conjunctivitis, alopecia, fatigue, arthralgias/myalgias, osteophytes, transient elevation of triglycerides
  * Bexarotene:
    * Phase II/III trial of 58 patients with relapsed stage IA–IIA disease showed 20% ORR at 6.5 mg/m^2, 54% at 300 mg/m^2, and 67% at 650 mg/m^2 daily dose, with median time to response of 8 weeks and median duration of response of 14, 30, and 74 weeks, respectively.[29]

- Phase II/III trial of 94 patients with relapsed stage IIB-IVB disease showed 45% ORR at 300 mg/m^2 and 55% ORR (13% CR) at 650 mg/m^2 daily dose.
  - Median time to response was 26 and 8 weeks, and duration of response was 43 and 55 weeks, respectively.
- Side effects: elevated triglycerides and cholesterol, central hypothyroidism, leucopenia, headache
  - Using HMG-coA reductase inhibitors and fenofibrate (but not gemfibrozil) for elevated triglycerides and cholesterol, as well as thyroid supplementation in cases of hypothyroidism is often necessary, helping to continue therapy.
- Daily dose of 300 mg/m2 balances response and toxicity.
- A small retrospective comparison of ATRA and bexarotene showed equivalent efficacy.[30]
- Retinoids can also be used with IFN or with PUVA, allowing a lower dose of both while maintaining the same efficacy.
- ECP
  - A way of administering PUVA systemically: patients undergo leukapheresis, white blood cells are mixed with 8-methoxypsoralen (8-MOP) and exposed to UVA ex vivo, then reinfused
  - Very effective for erythrodermic MF and SS
  - Initial multicenter study of 37 patients showed 73% ORR and 24% CR.
    - Response was seen in 24 of 29 patients with erythroderma, 8 of 10 with lymph node involvement, and 20 of 28 with resistance to standard chemotherapy.[31]
    - Follow-up suggested that ECP may prolong survival compared to historical controls (33 months vs. 60 months).[32]
  - Subsequent studies of 20 or more patients reported ORR of 31–80% and CR of 13–25%.
  - Side effects: hypotension, catheter-related complications
  - TSEBT followed by ECP: Wilson et al reported experience with 163 patients who had CR or good PR

with TSEBT and were offered adjuvant ECP or adriamycin with cyclophosphamide.

- Patients achieving CR with T1/2 disease did not benefit from adjuvant therapy, with OS of 85–90% at 5–10 years.
- Patients achieving CR with T3/4 disease benefited from adjuvant therapy: without adjuvant therapy OS was about 50% at 5 years, while it was 75% at 3 years with adjuvant adriamycin/cyclophosphamide and 100% at 3 years with ECP.[33]

- ECP can also be combined with IFN or with retinoids.
- Histone deacetylase inhibitors (vorinostat)
  - HDAC inhibitors allow transcription of genes related to cell cycle arrest and apoptosis.
  - First Food and Drug Administration (FDA) approved drug in the class is vorinostat (suberoylanilide hydroxamic acid).
  - Phase II trial in refractory CTCL where 8 of 33 (24%) patients achieved responses (all PRs), including 4 with SS.
    - Time to response was 2.7 months, duration of response was 3.5 months, and time to progression was 7.1 months.[34]
    - Of 3 dose schedules, 400 mg oral daily dose was selected for subsequent phase IIb trial.
  - Phase IIb trial enrolled 74 patients with stage IB-IVA (61 with stage IIB or above) persistent, progressive, or refractory disease.
    - 30% ORR: 30% in stage IIB and higher, 33% in SS patients; 1% CR
    - For all patients, median time to progression is 4.9 months.
    - For responders with stage IIB or above, median time to response is 1.8 months, median duration of response was at least 6.1 months and median time to progression was at least 9.8 months.[35]
  - Side effects: nausea/vomiting, diarrhea, fatigue, anorexia, thrombocytopenia (class effects)

- Denileukin diftitox
  - Interleukin 2-diphtheria toxin fusion protein
  - Pivotal phase III trial enrolled 71 patients with stage IB-IVA CTCL at 2 dosages
  - 30% ORR, 10% CR, median time to response 6 weeks, median duration of response 6.9 months[36]
  - Side effects: flu-like symptoms, acute infusion-related events, vascular leak syndrome (defined as at least 2 of: hypotension, edema, hypoalbuminemia), transaminitis
    - Incidence of vascular leak syndrome is reduced with intravenous fluids prior to drug administration
    - Incidence of flu-like symptoms is reduced with premedication (dexamethasone, diphenhydramine, acetaminophen)
  - Bexarotene was combined with denileukin diftitox, in a 14-patient phase I trial that showed 4 CRs and 4 PRs in 12 evaluable patients.[37]
- Single-agent chemotherapy
  - Methotrexate
    - Some efficacy in erythrodermic MF (T4) and early stage MF
      - Retrospective review of 29 patients treated with low-dose methotrexate (up to 75 mg weekly) showed 58% ORR and 41% CR, with median time to failure of 31 months.[38]
      - Similar review from the same group of 69 patients, 60 with T2 disease, showed lower ORR of 33% and CR of 12% with median time to failure of 15 months.[39]
      - Side effects: myelosuppression, gastrointestinal upset, oral mucositis
  - Gemcitabine
    - Pyrimidine analog, one of the most active agents in advanced CTCL
    - In 44 patients with relapsed disease (30 with MF), gemcitabine 1,200 mg/m^2 days 1,8, 15 of a 4-week cycle resulted in 70% ORR and 10% CR, with median CR duration of 15 months and median PR duration of 10 months.[40]

- Phase II trial in untreated patients (with 1,000 mg/m^2 on same schedule) showed similar ORR of 68% and CR of 8% in 31 patients, most with IIB–IVB.[41]
- Side effects: myelosuppression, hemolytic-uremic syndrome (in SS), mucositis, transaminitis
- Liposomal doxorubicin
  - Anthracyclines such as doxorubicin are very active in CTCL and improve CR rates as part of combination chemotherapy.
  - Pegylated liposomal formulation prolongs the half-life and alters the distribution of doxorubicin.
  - A multicenter retrospective study of 34 patients (27 receiving 20 mg/m^2 every 4 weeks) demonstrated 88% ORR and 44% CR, with median disease-free survival of 13 months and median OS of 18 months.[42]
  - A prospective phase II study of 19 patients confirmed high response, with 84% ORR, 42% CR, and suggested even better outcomes, with median progression-free survival (PFS) of 19 months and median OS of 34 months.[43]
  - Side effects: myelosuppression, hand-foot syndrome
- Purine nucleoside analogs (pentostatin, fludarabine, cladribine)
  - Pentostatin demonstrated the highest activity of the three agents.
    - Phase II trial of pentostatin in 42 patients from MD Anderson (32 with stage IIB-IV CTCL) showed 56% ORR and 13% CR in CTCL patients, with overall median duration of response of 4.3 months.[44]
    - Pentostatin + IFN: 41 patients, 41% ORR, 5% CR, median PFS of responders 13.1 months
      - No response in patients with visceral involvement
      - Significant infectious complications with herpes zoster and staphylococcal bacteremia[45]
  - Fludarabine:
    - 31 patients with stage III-IV disease were treated with 5-day course and showed only 19% ORR with 3% CR.[46]

- Fludarabine was followed by ECP consolidation in 19 of 44 patients in a study by Quaglino et al.
  - ORR in fludarabine + ECP group was higher (63% vs. 30%) but without a significant difference in time to progression (13 vs. 7 months).[47]
- Fludarabine + IFN: 35 patients, 51% ORR, 11% CR, with responses in 4 of 11 patients with visceral involvement, but median PFS of responders was only 5.9 months[48]
- Cladribine: largest study to date is a phase II trial by Kuzel et al in 21 patients with relapsed/refractory CTCL, showing 28% ORR, 14% CR, median CR duration of 4.5 months.[49]
- Several studies of purine analogs demonstrated a higher response in SS than in MF.
- Side effects: profound myelosuppression, opportunistic infections
  - Infectious complications reduced with anti-herpetic and anti-Pneumocystis jirovecii (PCP) pneumonia prophylaxis
- Chlorambucil with prednisone was used as principal treatment in 40 patients with SS by Winkelmann et al, and survival compared favorably to other therapies (median OS 6.2 vs 3.05 years).[50]
  - A small pilot of pulse-dose chlorambucil and a steroid fluocortolone showed responses in all 13 patients with erythrodermic MF (6 CRs), with median remission duration of 12 months.[51]
- Alemtuzumab
  - Humanized monoclonal antibody against CD52, present on malignant T and B cells
  - A phase II trial in advanced CTCL demonstrated 55% ORR, 32% CR, median time to treatment failure of 12 months, and cytomegalovirus (CMV) reactivation in 18% of the patients.[52]
  - Side effects: infusion reactions with IV administration, lymphopenia, opportunistic infections (particularly CMV reactivation)
- Combination chemotherapy:
  - Combination chemotherapy may achieve faster remission onset and higher remission rates, but has

similar duration of remission (usually less than a year) with more toxicity (such as myelosuppression and infections) as compared to single-agent chemotherapy.

- The largest trial by Kaye et al randomized 103 patients to either 30 Gy of TSEBT plus combination chemotherapy (cyclophosphamide, doxorubicine, vincristine, etoposide), or to sequential topical treatments.
  - Combination therapy resulted in significantly higher CR rates (38% vs. 18%, p=0.032) but also had more complications, including 2 cases of acute myelogenous leukemia.
  - There was no difference in DFS or OS.[53]
- CHOP-like regimens:
  - An earlier trial from Southwest Oncology Group reported the results of 3 regimens in 24 patients with CTCL: CHOP (n=7), HOP (CHOP without cyclophosphamide) (n=5), and COP-bleomycin (CHOP without doxorubicin) (n=12).
    - ORR was 95% with 29% CR and median OS of 95 weeks.
    - Doxorubicin-containing chemotherapy was associated with a higher CR rate but COP-bleomycin was associated with a longer median duration of remission.[54]
  - A more contemporary study showed 40% ORR and 23% CR in 35 patients with CTCL.
    - Median response duration was 5.7 months and median OS was 19 months.[55]
- Transplantation:
  - Autologous stem cell transplantation (ASCT) performed in a pilot study with 9 patients resulted in 1 death from septicemia and CR in the others.
    - Remissions were short—7 of 8 relapsed at a median of 7 months.[56]
  - Allogeneic stem cell transplantation (AlloSCT) resulted in complete remission in all 8 patients with heavily pretreated CTCL in a retrospective review, but 2 patients died from treatment-related complications.[57]

- ASCT appears to be of limited value as compared to combination chemotherapy, while AlloSCT demonstrates some graft-vs.-lymphoma effect and may be tried in highly refractory CTCL.

◾ General Treatment Approach

Also see National Comprehensive Cancer Network recommendations (http://www.nccn.org/professionals/physician_gls/PDF/nhl.pdf), as well as European Organisation for Research and Treatment of Cancer guidelines.[58]

- IA (T1): any skin-directed therapy; in relapse use a different topical therapy
- IB/IIA (T2): skin-directed therapy (chemotherapy, phototherapy, or TSEBT); in relapse may also use oral retinoids, denileukin diftitox, or IFN
- IIB (T3): any two of three (PUVA, oral retinoid, and IFN), TSEBT; in relapse, denileukin diftitox, vorinostat, or single agent chemotherapy
  - Combine with skin-directed therapy as needed.
  - Folliculotropic and transformed MF treated similarly
- III (T4): IFN, oral retinoid, ECP, vorinostat, denileukin diftitox, methotrexate; in relapse, may combine ECP + oral retinoid or IFN, single agent chemotherapy
  - Combine with skin-directed therapy as needed.
- IV (N2–3/M): single agent chemotherapy (e.g., gemcitabine, liposomal doxorubicin, chlorambucil + prednisone, methotrexate, vorinostat), alemtuzumab, oral retinoid, denileukin diftitox, IFN
  - Combine with skin-directed therapy as needed.
  - With bulky lymph nodes consider adding radiation therapy.
  - With blood involvement, use ECP + oral retinoid or IFN.
- SS: ECP, IFN, denileukin diftitox; if relapsed, oral retinoids, single agent chemotherapy (e.g., gemcitabine, liposomal doxorubicin, chlorambucil + prednisone, methotrexate)
  - Combine with skin-directed therapy as needed.

■ MF Variants

Folliculotropic MF

■ Atypical T-cells surround the hair follicles, without epidermotropism.

■ Frequent destruction of the follicles with mucin (follicular mucinosis)

■ Acne-like lesions, most prominently affecting head and neck

■ Associated with alopecia, including eyebrows

■ Usually presents at T1 or T2 stage but has worse prognosis as compared to the same stage of classic MF, more similar to T3

   • Largest case series followed 51 patients, 82% male, with only 27% having nodules/tumors at diagnosis.

   • DFS was 68% at 5 years and 26% at 10 years.[59]

■ May be less responsive to localized (skin-directed) therapies due to the deep location of the infiltrate[1]

■ Treatment: radiation (EBT, TSEBT), retinoids, interferon, +/− PUVA

Pagetoid Reticulosis (Workinger-Kolopp Disease)

■ Very rare

■ Presents as single scaly crusted patch or plaque, usually on an extremity

■ Progresses slowly, does not disseminate, with excellent prognosis

■ Pathology shows atypical pagetoid lymphocytes infiltrating the epidermal layer only (hence pagetoid).

■ Unlike other types of MF, neoplastic T-cells may be CD4+ or CD8+.[1]

■ Treatment: radiation or excision

Granulomatous Slack Skin

■ Extremely rare (fewer than 100 cases reported)

■ Large skin folds develop in groin and axilla

■ Pathology often shows many multinucleated giant cells.

■ One-third associated with Hodgkin's lymphoma, some with classic MF[1]

- Indolent but progressive course
- Treatment difficult to define due to rarity, but radiation often attempted

■ References

1. Willemze R, Jaffe ES, Burg G, et al. WHO-EORTC classification for cutaneous lymphomas. *Blood.* 2005;105(10):3768–3785.

2. Scheffer E, Meijer CJ, Van Vloten WA. Dermatopathic lymphadenopathy and lymph node involvement in mycosis fungoides. *Cancer.* 1980;45(1):137–148.

3. Clendenning WE, Rappaport HW. Report of the Committee on Pathology of Cutaneous T Cell Lymphomas. *Cancer Treat Rep.* 1979;63(4):719–724.

4. Jaffe ES, Harris NL, Stein H, Vardiman JW. *World Health Organization Classification of Tumours: Pathology and Genetics of Tumours of Haematopoietic and Lymphoid Tissues.* Lyon: IARC Press; 2001.

5. Sterry W. Cutaneous T-cell lymphoma: molecular and cytogenetic findings. *Oncology (Williston Park).* 2007;21(2 Suppl 1): 13–17.

6. Tracey L, Villuendas R, Dotor AM, et al. Mycosis fungoides shows concurrent deregulation of multiple genes involved in the TNF signaling pathway: an expression profile study. *Blood.* 2003;102(3):1042–1050.

7. Kari L, Loboda A, Nebozhyn M, et al. Classification and prediction of survival in patients with the leukemic phase of cutaneous T cell lymphoma. *J Exp Med.* 2003;197(11): 1477–1488.

8. Bunn PA, Jr., Lamberg SI. Report of the Committee on Staging and Classification of Cutaneous T-Cell Lymphomas. *Cancer Treat Rep.* 1979;63(4):725–728.

9. Olsen E, Vonderheid E, Pimpinelli N, et al. Revisions to the staging and classification of mycosis fungoides and Sézary syndrome: a proposal of the International Society for Cutaneous Lymphomas (ISCL) and the Cutaneous Lymphoma Task Force of the European Organization of Research and Treatment of Cancer (EORTC). *Blood.* 2007; 110(6):1713–1722.

10. de Coninck EC, Kim YH, Varghese A, Hoppe RT. Clinical characteristics and outcome of patients with extracutaneous mycosis fungoides. *J Clin Oncol.* 2001;19(3):779–784.

10a. Kim YH, Liu HL, Mraz-Gernhard S, et al. Long-term outcome of 525 patients with mycosis fungoides and Sézary syndrome. *Arch Dermatol.* Jul 2003;139:857–866.

11. Vonderheid EC, Bernengo MG, Burg G, et al. Update on erythrodermic cutaneous T-cell lymphoma: report of the International Society for Cutaneous Lymphomas. *J Am Acad Dermatol.* 2002;46(1):95–106.

12. Duvic M, Olsen EA, Omura GA, et al. A phase III, randomized, double-blind, placebo-controlled study of peldesine (BCX-34) cream as topical therapy for cutaneous T-cell lymphoma. *J Am Acad Dermatol.* 2001;44(6):940–947.

13. Duvic M, Hymes K, Heald P, et al. Bexarotene is effective and safe for treatment of refractory advanced-stage cutaneous T-cell lymphoma: multinational phase II-III trial results. *J Clin Oncol.* 2001;19(9):2456–2471.

14. Zackheim HS, Kashani-Sabet M, Amin S. Topical corticosteroids for mycosis fungoides. Experience in 79 patients. *Arch Dermatol.* 1998;134(8):949–954.

15. Kim YH, Martinez G, Varghese A, Hoppe RT. Topical nitrogen mustard in the management of mycosis fungoides: update of the Stanford experience. *Arch Dermatol.* 2003; 139(2):165–173.

16. Zackheim HS, Epstein EH, Jr., Crain WR. Topical carmustine (BCNU) for cutaneous T cell lymphoma: a 15-year experience in 143 patients. *J Am Acad Dermatol.* 1990; 22(5 Pt 1): 802–810.

17. Breneman D, Duvic M, Kuzel T, Yocum R, Truglia J, Stevens VJ. Phase 1 and 2 trial of bexarotene gel for skin-directed treatment of patients with cutaneous T-cell lymphoma. *Arch Dermatol.* 2002;138(3):325–332.

18. Apisarnthanarax N, Talpur R, Ward S, Ni X, Kim HW, Duvic M. Tazarotene 0.1% gel for refractory mycosis fungoides lesions: an open-label pilot study. *J Am Acad Dermatol.* 2004;50(4):600–607.

19. Roenigk HH, Jr., Kuzel TM, Skoutelis AP, et al. Photochemotherapy alone or combined with interferon alpha-2a in the treatment of cutaneous T-cell lymphoma. *J Invest Dermatol.* 1990;95(6 Suppl):198S–205S.

20. Herrmann JJ, Roenigk HH, Jr., Hurria A, et al. Treatment of mycosis fungoides with photochemotherapy (PUVA): long-term follow-up. *J Am Acad Dermatol.* 1995;33(2 Pt 1):234–242.

21. Querfeld C, Rosen ST, Kuzel TM, et al. Long-term follow-up of patients with early-stage cutaneous T-cell lymphoma

who achieved complete remission with psoralen plus UV-A monotherapy. *Arch Dermatol.* 2005;141(3):305–311.

22. Ramsay DL, Lish KM, Yalowitz CB, Soter NA. Ultraviolet-B phototherapy for early-stage cutaneous T-cell lymphoma. *Arch Dermatol.* 1992;128(7):931–933.

23. Diederen PV, van Weelden H, Sanders CJ, Toonstra J, van Vloten WA. Narrowband UVB and psoralen-UVA in the treatment of early-stage mycosis fungoides: a retrospective study. *J Am Acad Dermatol.* 2003;48(2):215–219.

24. Cotter GW, Baglan RJ, Wasserman TH, Mill W. Palliative radiation treatment of cutaneous mycosis fungoides—a dose response. *Int J Radiat Oncol Biol Phys.* 1983;9(10):1477–1480.

25. Jones GW, Hoppe RT, Glatstein E. Electron beam treatment for cutaneous T-cell lymphoma. *Hematol Oncol Clin North Am.* 1995;9(5):1057–1076.

26. Hamminga B, Noordijk EM, van Vloten WA. Treatment of mycosis fungoides: total-skin electron-beam irradiation vs topical mechlorethamine therapy. *Arch Dermatol.* 1982;118(3):150–153.

27. Kuzel TM, Roenigk HH, Jr., Samuelson E, et al. Effectiveness of interferon alfa-2a combined with phototherapy for mycosis fungoides and the Sézary syndrome. *J Clin Oncol.* 1995;13(1):257–263.

28. Kaplan EH, Rosen ST, Norris DB, Roenigk HH, Jr., Saks SR, Bunn PA, Jr. Phase II study of recombinant human interferon gamma for treatment of cutaneous T-cell lymphoma. *J Natl Cancer Inst.* 1990;82(3):208–212.

29. Duvic M, Martin AG, Kim Y, et al. Phase 2 and 3 clinical trial of oral bexarotene (Targretin capsules) for the treatment of refractory or persistent early-stage cutaneous T-cell lymphoma. *Arch Dermatol.* 2001;137(5):581–593.

30. Querfeld C, Rosen ST, Guitart J, et al. Comparison of selective retinoic acid receptor- and retinoic X receptor-mediated efficacy, tolerance, and survival in cutaneous t-cell lymphoma. *J Am Acad Dermatol.* 2004;51(1):25–32.

31. Edelson R, Berger C, Gasparro F, et al. Treatment of cutaneous T-cell lymphoma by extracorporeal photochemotherapy. Preliminary results. *N Engl J Med.* 1987;316(6): 297–303.

32. Heald P, Rook A, Perez M, et al. Treatment of erythrodermic cutaneous T-cell lymphoma with extracorporeal photochemotherapy. *J Am Acad Dermatol.* 1992;27(3):427–433.

33. Wilson LD, Licata AL, Braverman IM, et al. Systemic chemotherapy and extracorporeal photochemotherapy for

T3 and T4 cutaneous T-cell lymphoma patients who have achieved a complete response to total skin electron beam therapy. *Int J Radiat Oncol Biol Phys.* 1995;32(4):987–995.

34.   Duvic M, Talpur R, Ni X, et al. Phase 2 trial of oral vorinostat (suberoylanilide hydroxamic acid, SAHA) for refractory cutaneous T-cell lymphoma (CTCL). *Blood.* 2007;109(1): 31–39.

35.   Olsen EA, Kim YH, Kuzel TM, et al. Phase IIb multicenter trial of vorinostat in patients with persistent, progressive, or treatment refractory cutaneous T-cell lymphoma. *J Clin Oncol.* 2007;25(21):3109–3115.

36.   Olsen E, Duvic M, Frankel A, et al. Pivotal phase III trial of two dose levels of denileukin diftitox for the treatment of cutaneous T-cell lymphoma. *J Clin Oncol.* 2001;19(2):376–388.

37.   Foss F, Demierre MF, DiVenuti G. A phase-1 trial of bexarotene and denileukin diftitox in patients with relapsed or refractory cutaneous T-cell lymphoma. *Blood.* 2005; 106(2):454–457.

38.   Zackheim HS, Kashani-Sabet M, Hwang ST. Low-dose methotrexate to treat erythrodermic cutaneous T-cell lymphoma: results in twenty-nine patients. *J Am Acad Dermatol.* 1996;34(4):626–631.

39.   Zackheim HS, Kashani-Sabet M, McMillan A. Low-dose methotrexate to treat mycosis fungoides: a retrospective study in 69 patients. *J Am Acad Dermatol.* 2003;49(5):873–878.

40.   Zinzani PL, Baliva G, Magagnoli M, et al. Gemcitabine treatment in pretreated cutaneous T-cell lymphoma: experience in 44 patients. *J Clin Oncol.* 2000;18(13):2603–2606.

41.   Duvic M, Talpur R, Wen S, Kurzrock R, David CL, Apisarnthanarax N. Phase II evaluation of gemcitabine monotherapy for cutaneous T-cell lymphoma. *Clin Lymphoma Myeloma.* 2006;7(1):51–58.

42.   Wollina U, Dummer R, Brockmeyer NH, et al. Multicenter study of pegylated liposomal doxorubicin in patients with cutaneous T-cell lymphoma. *Cancer.* 2003;98(5):993–1001.

43.   Pulini S, Rupoli S, Goteri G, et al. Pegylated liposomal doxorubicin in the treatment of primary cutaneous T-cell lymphomas. *Haematologica.* 2007;92(5):686–689.

44.   Tsimberidou AM, Giles F, Duvic M, Fayad L, Kurzrock R. Phase II study of pentostatin in advanced T-cell lymphoid malignancies: update of an M.D. Anderson Cancer Center series. *Cancer.* 2004;100(2):342–349.

45.   Foss FM, Ihde DC, Breneman DL, et al. Phase II study of pentostatin and intermittent high-dose recombinant

interferon alfa-2a in advanced mycosis fungoides/Sézary syndrome. *J Clin Oncol.* 1992;10(12):1907–1913.

46. Von Hoff DD, Dahlberg S, Hartstock RJ, Eyre HJ. Activity of fludarabine monophosphate in patients with advanced mycosis fungoides: a Southwest Oncology Group study. *J Natl Cancer Inst.* 1990;82(16):1353–1355.

47. Quaglino P, Fierro MT, Rossotto GL, Savoia P, Bernengo MG. Treatment of advanced mycosis fungoides/Sézary syndrome with fludarabine and potential adjunctive benefit to subsequent extracorporeal photochemotherapy. *Br J Dermatol.* 2004;150(2):327–336.

48. Foss FM, Ihde DC, Linnoila IR, et al. Phase II trial of fludarabine phosphate and interferon alfa-2a in advanced mycosis fungoides/Sézary syndrome. *J Clin Oncol.* 1994;12(10): 2051–2059.

49. Kuzel TM, Hurria A, Samuelson E, et al. Phase II trial of 2-chlorodeoxyadenosine for the treatment of cutaneous T-cell lymphoma. *Blood.* 1996;87(3):906–911.

50. Winkelmann RK, Diaz-Perez JL, Buechner SA. The treatment of Sézary syndrome. *J Am Acad Dermatol.* 1984;10(6): 1000–1004.

51. Coors EA, von den Driesch P. Treatment of erythrodermic cutaneous T-cell lymphoma with intermittent chlorambucil and fluocortolone therapy. *Br J Dermatol.* 2000;143(1): 127–131.

52. Lundin J, Hagberg H, Repp R, et al. Phase 2 study of alemtuzumab (anti-CD52 monoclonal antibody) in patients with advanced mycosis fungoides/Sézary syndrome. *Blood.* 2003; 101(11):4267–4272.

53. Kaye FJ, Bunn PA, Jr., Steinberg SM, et al. A randomized trial comparing combination electron-beam radiation and chemotherapy with topical therapy in the initial treatment of mycosis fungoides. *N Engl J Med.* 1989;321(26):1784–1790.

54. Grozea PN, Jones SE, McKelvey EM, Coltman CA, Jr., Fisher R, Haskins CL. Combination chemotherapy for mycosis fungoides: a Southwest Oncology Group study. *Cancer Treat Rep.* 1979;63(4):647–653.

55. Fierro MT, Quaglino P, Savoia P, Verrone A, Bernengo MG. Systemic polychemotherapy in the treatment of primary cutaneous lymphomas: a clinical follow-up study of 81 patients treated with COP or CHOP. *Leuk Lymphoma.* 1998; 31(5–6):583–588.

56.   Olavarria E, Child F, Woolford A, et al. T-cell depletion and autologous stem cell transplantation in the management of tumour stage mycosis fungoides with peripheral blood involvement. *Br J Haematol.* 2001;114(3):624–631.

57.   Molina A, Zain J, Arber DA, et al. Durable clinical, cytogenetic, and molecular remissions after allogeneic hematopoietic cell transplantation for refractory Sézary syndrome and mycosis fungoides. *J Clin Oncol.* 2005;23(25):6163–6171.

58.   Trautinger F, Knobler R, Willemze R, et al. EORTC consensus recommendations for the treatment of mycosis fungoides/Sézary syndrome. *Eur J Cancer.* 2006;42(8):1014–1030.

59.   van Doorn R, Scheffer E, Willemze R. Follicular mycosis fungoides, a distinct disease entity with or without associated follicular mucinosis: a clinicopathologic and follow-up study of 51 patients. *Arch Dermatol.* 2002;138(2):191–198.

Index

Note: Page numbers with *f* indicate figures, *t* indicate tables.

A

AAIPI (age-adjusted International Prognostic Index), 22–24
ABC (activated B-cell-like) phenotype, 21
abdominal mass, 6, 157
ABVD (doxorubicin, bleomycin, vinblastine, and dacarbazine), 55–56
  for HL, advanced, 115–120, 122, 142
  for HL, early, 112–114
  for HL, relapsed or refractory, 127
  regimen, 141
  secondary disease following, 129, 130
acute myelogenous leukemia (AML), 50, 116
ACVBP (doxorubicin, cyclophosphamide, vindesine, bleomycin, and prednisone), for DLBCL, 28
adenopathy, cervical, 5. *See also* lymphadenopathy
Adriamycin. *See* doxorubicin
Age. *See also* presentation *and specific lymphomas*
  average at presentation, summary, 11
  and DLBCL prognosis, 22–24
  and HL prognosis, 107–110
  incidence and, 1
  and splenic MZL, 76
aggressive lymphomas, 12
  chemotherapy regimens, 146–150

clinical behavior, 12
listing of, 12
presentation, 2
risk factors and prognosis, 22–23
staging, 13
alemtuxumab, 180
ALK-1 antibody analysis, 7, 8
alkylators
  multiagent
    for extranodal MZL, advanced, 79
    for FL, advanced or relapsed, 51
    for splenic MZL, advanced, 78, 80
  secondary disease following, 50, 128, 129
  single-agent
    for FL, advanced or relapsed, 50–51
    for MZL of MAST, advanced or relapsed, 74
allogeneic transplantation (allo-transplant)
  DLBCL, relapsed or refractory, 33
  FL, 47, 59–60
  HL, relapsed or refractory, 125–126
  MCL, 94–95
alpha-chain disease (MZL variant), 75
AML (acute myelogenous leukemia), 50, 116
anaplastic large cell lymphoma (primary systemic). *See also* DLBCL

193

CPSIA information can be obtained at www.ICGtesting.com
231075LV00004B/17/P

9 780763 750244